Chef Michael's Table

The Spirit of Food and Family

Chef Michael Gattis

PASTA WITH RED CRAB SAUCE

INGREDIENTS

For the Crab Stock:
- 8-10 blue crab shells (or any other crab shells available)
- 2 tbsp olive oil
- 1 large onion, roughly chopped
- 2 celery stalks, roughly chopped
- 1 large carrot, roughly chopped
- 4 garlic cloves, smashed
- 1/2 cup dry white wine
- 4 cups water
- 1 bay leaf
- Fresh parsley stems
- Salt and pepper, to taste

For the Sauce:
- 1/4 cup olive oil
- 1 medium onion, finely diced
- 2-3 garlic cloves, minced
- 1/4 tsp red pepper flakes (optional, for a hint of heat)
- 1/2 cup dry white wine
- 1 can (28 oz) whole peeled tomatoes, crushed by hand
- Fresh basil leaves (about 5-6 large leaves), torn
- 2 tbsp fresh parsley, finely chopped
- 1 lb fresh crab meat (or cooked, shelled crab meat)
- Salt and pepper, to taste

For the Pasta:
- 1 lb spaghetti or linguine
- Salt for the pasta water

Garnish:
- Fresh parsley, finely chopped
- Extra basil leaves
- Freshly grated Parmesan cheese (optional)
- Lemon wedges for serving

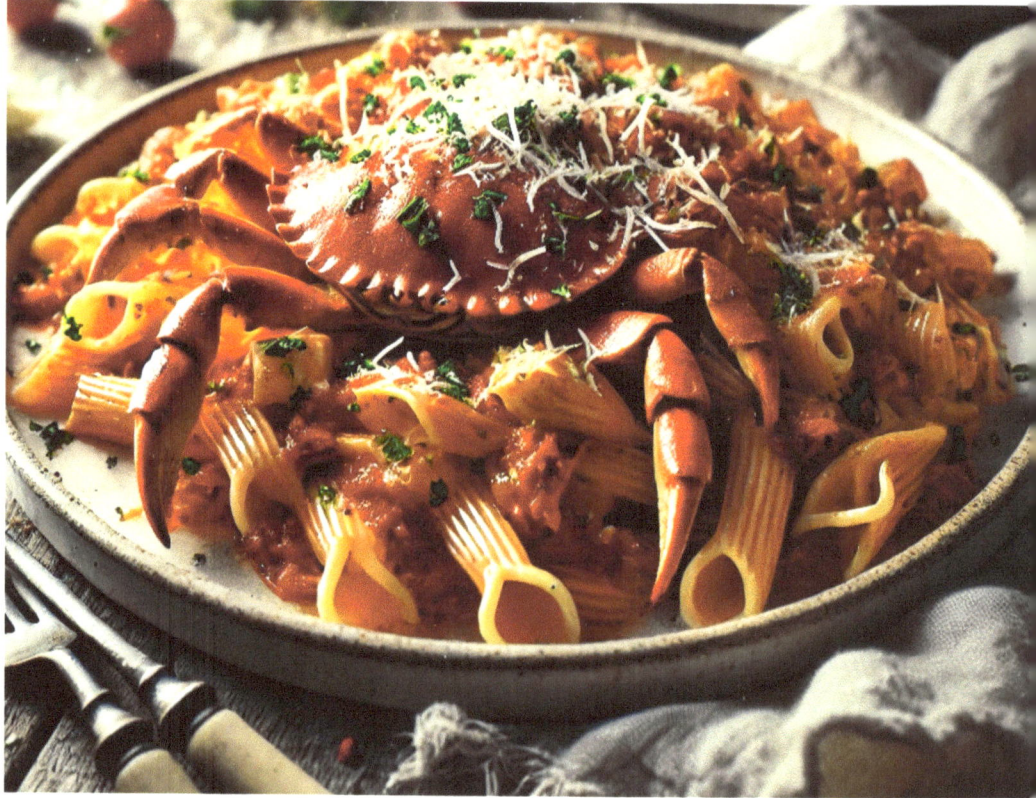

DIRECTIONS

STEP 1
PREPARE THE CRAB STOCK

1 **Heat the Oil:** In a large stockpot, heat the olive oil over medium heat. Add the crab shells and sauté for about 5 minutes, stirring occasionally, until they turn a bright red color and release their aroma.
2 **Add Vegetables:** Add the chopped onion, celery, carrot, and garlic to the pot. Sauté for another 5 minutes until the vegetables start to soften.
3 **Deglaze and Simmer:** Pour in the white wine to deglaze the pot, scraping up any browned bits from the bottom. Let the wine cook down by about half, then add water, bay leaf, parsley stems, salt, and pepper.
4 **Simmer the Stock:** Bring the mixture to a gentle boil, then reduce the heat to low. Simmer for 30-40 minutes to develop a rich, flavorful broth.
5 **Strain:** Once done, strain the stock through a fine sieve into a bowl and discard the solids. Set the stock aside to use in the sauce.

STEP 2
MAKE THE CRAB SAUCE

1 **Saute the Onion ,Crab and Garlic:** In a large skillet, heat olive oil over medium heat. Add diced onion and cleaned crabs, sauté 4-5 minutes until red and fragrant, add minced garlic and cook another 1-2 minutes.
2 **Add Red Pepper and Deglaze:** Add red pepper flakes for a touch of heat (if using) and pour in the white wine. Allow it to simmer for 2-3 minutes, reducing slightly.
3 **Add Tomatoes and Stock:** Add the crushed tomatoes and about 1 to 1 1/2 cups of the reserved crab stock. Stir well to combine.
4 **Simmer and Season:** Bring the sauce to a gentle simmer. Add torn basil leaves, chopped parsley, and season with salt and pepper. Let it simmer uncovered for 15-20 minutes, stirring occasionally, until the sauce thickens slightly.
5 **Add Crab Meat:** Gently fold in the fresh crab meat, stirring carefully to avoid breaking up large pieces. Allow the crab to heat through in the sauce for about 5 minutes. Taste and adjust seasoning if necessary.

STEP 3
COOK THE PASTA

1 **Boil the Pasta:** Bring a large pot of salted water to a boil. Add the pasta and cook according to package instructions until al dente. Reserve about 1/2 cup of pasta water, then drain the pasta.
2 **Combine Pasta and Sauce:** Add the cooked pasta to the skillet with the sauce, tossing gently to coat each strand. If the sauce is too thick, add a bit of the reserved pasta water to loosen it.

STEP 4
SERVE

1 **Plate the Pasta:** Serve the pasta in shallow bowls, making sure to add plenty of sauce and crab meat to each plate.
2 **Garnish:** Top with freshly chopped parsley, additional basil leaves, and, if desired, a sprinkle of Parmesan cheese.
3 **Add Lemon and Enjoy:** Serve with lemon wedges on the side to squeeze over the pasta for a hint of acidity that complements the crab.

FRESH MOZZARELLA FROM CURD RECIPE

Making fresh mozzarella from curd is a fun, hands-on process that requires some precision but is well worth it for the fresh, creamy cheese you'll produce. Here's a detailed recipe to guide you through making mozzarella from mozzarella curd.

INGREDIENTS

- 1 lb mozzarella curd (typically available at specialty cheese shops or Italian markets)
- 1/4 cup kosher salt
- 8 cups water (divided into separate bowls for heating and cooling)

EQUIPMENT NEEDED

- Large mixing bowl
- Slotted spoon
- Thermometer
- Rubber gloves (optional, for handling hot curds)

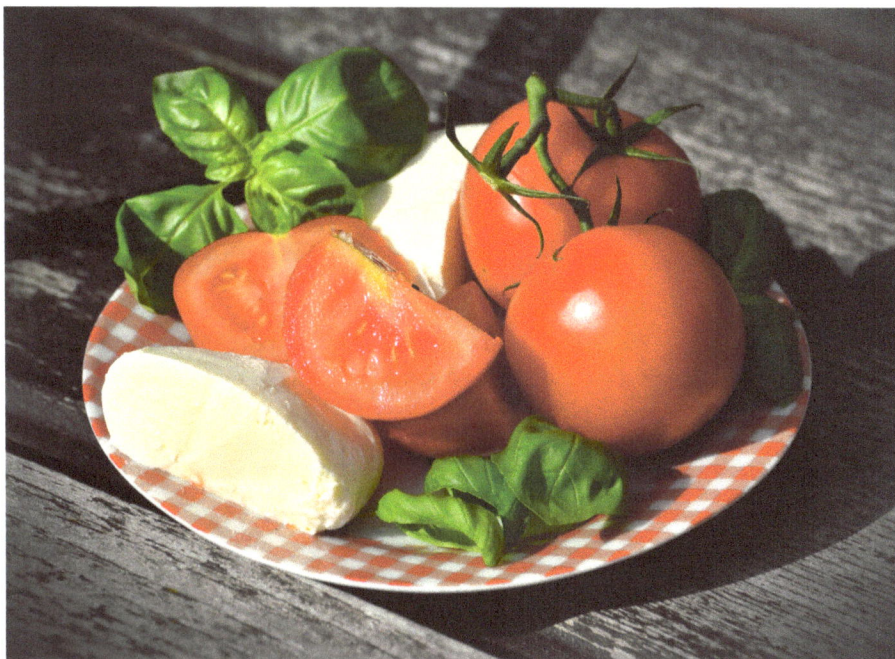

DIRECTIONS

STEP 1
PREPARE THE WATER

1 **Salted Water for Heating:** In a large pot, heat 4 cups of water to about 170°F (76°C). Dissolve the salt into the water, stirring well.
2 **Cool Water Bath:** In a separate bowl, prepare a cool water bath with 4 cups of room temperature water. This will be used to cool and set the cheese.

STEP 2
CUT AND PREPARE THE CURD

1 **Cut the Curd:** Slice the mozzarella curd into small, bite-sized cubes (about 1-2 inches each). This allows the heat to evenly distribute, making it easier to stretch the curd.
2 **Place in Bowl:** Put the curd pieces into a large mixing bowl, making sure they're evenly spread out.

STEP 3
HEAT AND SOFTEN THE CURD

1 **Add Hot Salted Water:** Pour the heated salted water over the curds in the bowl, ensuring that they're fully submerged. Let them sit for a few minutes until they soften and start to melt slightly.
2 **Check Temperature:** The water should remain around 160-170°F (71-76°C) to keep the curd pliable. If needed, add more hot water to maintain the temperature.

STEP 4
STRETCHING THE MOZZARELLA

1 **Begin Stretching:** Using a slotted spoon or gloved hands, lift the softened curds and start gently folding and stretching them. Continue this motion until the curd becomes smooth and glossy. Avoid overstretching, which can make the mozzarella tough.
2 **Fold and Stretch:** Stretch the cheese gently, folding it over itself. You'll notice it becomes more elastic and smooth as it stretches, which is the desired texture for mozzarella.
3 **Form into Balls:** Once you have a glossy, stretchy consistency, shape the mozzarella into small balls or one large ball, depending on your preference.

STEP 5
SET THE CHEESE

1 **Cool in Water Bath:** Immediately place the shaped mozzarella balls in the bowl of cool water to set their shape and texture.
2 **Optional Final Salt Bath:** For additional seasoning, briefly place the mozzarella in a fresh salted water bath to add a final touch of flavor.

STEP 6
SERVE AND ENJOY

1 **Serve Fresh:** Mozzarella is best enjoyed fresh. Serve it with sliced tomatoes, fresh basil, a drizzle of olive oil, and a balsamic reduction for a classic caprese appetizer, or enjoy it as a topping on pizza or in any dish where you want fresh, gooey cheese.

GARLIC SHRIMP APPETIZER WITH SHRIMP SHELL STOCK SAUCE

INGREDIENTS

Shrimp and Garlic Sauce

- 1 lb large shrimp (peeled and deveined, with shells reserved)
- 5 cloves garlic, thinly sliced
- 3 tbsp olive oil
- 1/4 cup white wine (dry)
- 1 tbsp fresh lemon juice
- 2 tbsp unsalted butter
- Salt and pepper to taste
- Fresh parsley, chopped, for garnish

Shrimp Shell Stock

- Shrimp shells from 1 lb of shrimp
- 1/2 small onion, roughly chopped
- 1 small carrot, roughly chopped
- 1 celery stalk, roughly chopped
- 1 clove garlic, crushed
- 2 cups water
- 1 bay leaf
- 1/4 tsp black peppercorns

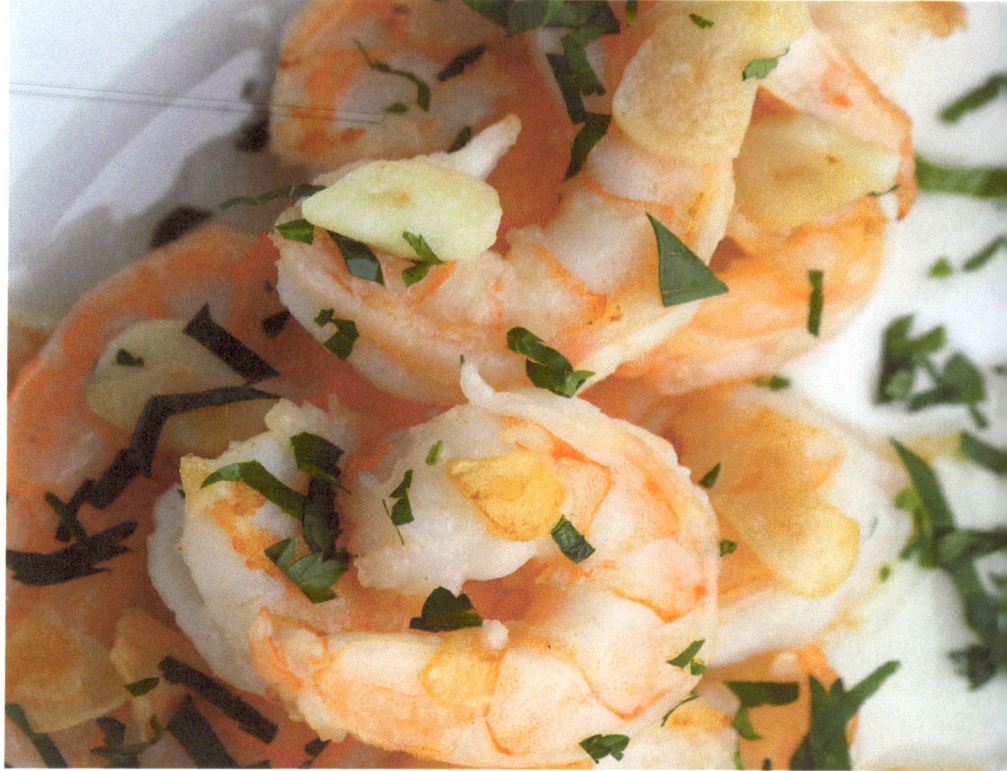

DIRECTIONS

STEP 1
MAKE THE SHRIMP SHELL STOCK

1. **Prepare Shrimp Shells:** In a medium saucepan, heat a tablespoon of olive oil over medium heat. Add the reserved shrimp shells and cook for 2-3 minutes, stirring occasionally, until they turn pink and start to release their aroma.
2. **Add Vegetables:** Add the chopped onion, carrot, celery, and crushed garlic to the pan. Sauté the mixture for another 3-4 minutes, until the vegetables start to soften.
3. **Add Water and Seasoning:** Pour in 2 cups of water, add the bay leaf and black peppercorns, and bring to a boil. Reduce the heat and simmer uncovered for 20-25 minutes, allowing the flavors to develop.
4. **Strain the Stock:** After simmering, strain the stock through a fine-mesh sieve, discarding the solids. Reserve about 1/2 cup of the stock for the garlic shrimp sauce.

STEP 2
COOK THE GARLIC SHRIMP

1. **Prepare the Pan:** In a large skillet, heat 3 tablespoons of olive oil over medium-low heat. Add the sliced garlic and cook gently, stirring frequently, until the garlic is golden and fragrant. Be careful not to let it burn, as burnt garlic can become bitter.
2. **Sauté the Shrimp:** Increase the heat to medium. Add the shrimp to the pan and cook for 1-2 minutes on each side, until they just turn pink. Remove the shrimp and set aside on a plate, leaving the garlic and oil in the pan.
3. **Deglaze with White Wine:** Pour the white wine into the skillet, stirring to deglaze any browned bits from the bottom of the pan. Let the wine reduce by half, which will take about 2-3 minutes.
4. **Add the Shrimp Stock:** Pour in 1/2 cup of the reserved shrimp stock, along with the lemon juice. Let the mixture simmer and reduce slightly for 3-4 minutes.

STEP 3
FINISH THE SAUCE

1. **Finish with Butter:** Lower the heat to medium-low and whisk in the butter, letting it melt into the sauce. Stir until the sauce is smooth and slightly thickened.
2. **Return the Shrimp:** Add the shrimp back into the skillet, along with any juices that have collected on the plate. Cook for an additional 1-2 minutes, tossing to coat the shrimp in the sauce. Season with salt and pepper to taste.

STEP 4
SERVE

1. **Plate the Dish:** Transfer the garlic shrimp to a serving dish, drizzle with any remaining sauce, and sprinkle with freshly chopped parsley.
2. **Optional:** Serve with crusty bread on the side for dipping.

TIPS

- **Using the Stock:** The homemade shrimp shell stock enhances the depth of the sauce, creating a rich, seafood-forward flavor.
- **Garlic Levels:** For even more garlic intensity, feel free to increase the amount, or alternatively, roast the garlic separately for a sweeter flavor

WIELGUS FAMILY WALNUT LOAF

INGREDIENTS

For The Slovak Kolache Dough
- 3 tsp active dry yeast
- ½ cup milk, heated to 110° F
- ½ cup +1 teaspoon sugar, divided
- 1 tsp salt
- 1 cup butter, softened at room temperature
- 1 cup sour cream
- 3 eggs , beaten
- 5 cups all-purpose flour, plus more as needed

For The Walnut Filling
- 4 cups ground walnuts
- ¼ cup milk
- 2¼ tbsp butter, melted
- 1 cup sugar
- 1¼ tsp cinnamon

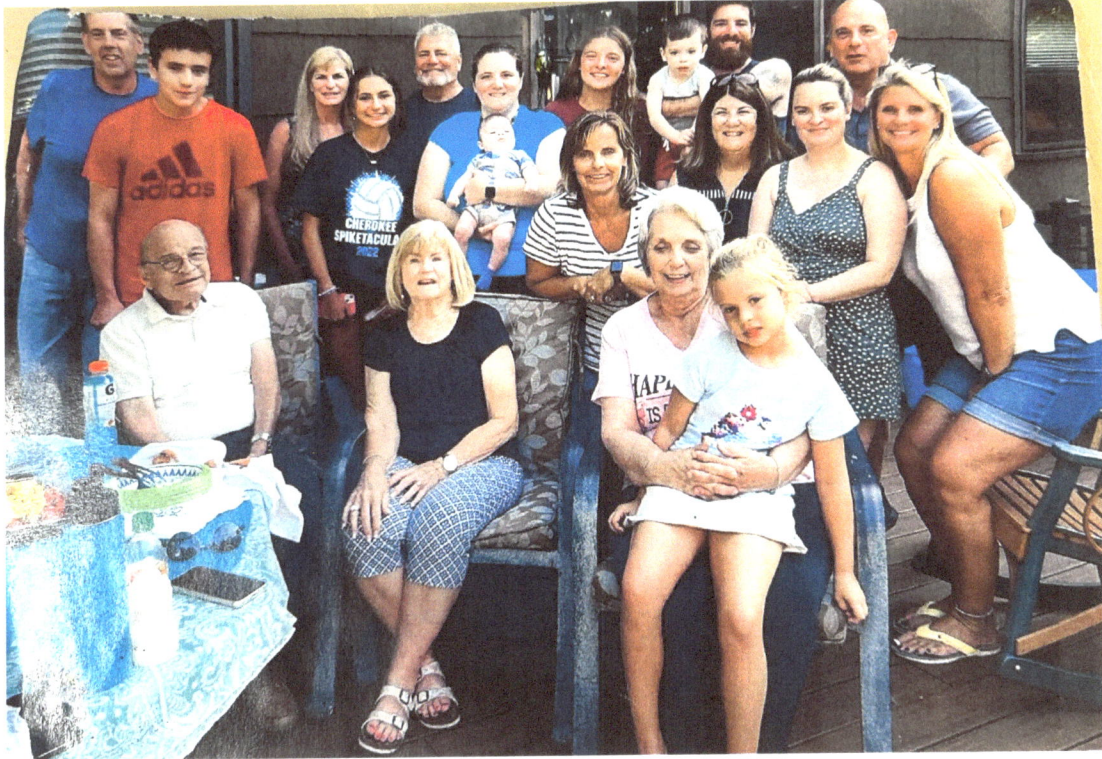

INSTRUCTIONS

Make the Filling
1. In a medium bowl, mix together the ground walnuts, milk, sugar, butter, and cinnamon until it forms a paste. Set aside.

Make the Slovak Kolache
1. In a small bowl. dissolve the yeast and 1 teaspoon sugar in the warm milk.
2. Using a stand mixer with a dough hook attachment, mix together the yeast mixture, remaining sugar, salt, butter, eggs, and sour cream. Beat on a low speed for a minute, then add the flour. Continue mixing on low for 2-3 minutes, then on medium-high for 5-6 minutes. The dough should be just slightly sticky. If needed, add another ½ cup of flour.
3. Form the dough into a ball, then transfer it to a greased bowl. Cover with cling wrap or cloth and allow the dough to rise in a warm place for 60-75 minutes, or until the dough has doubled.
4. Once the dough has doubled, punch it down with your fist, then divide into 3 equal pieces and roll each piece into a rectangle, about 1/a inch thick.
5. Brush each rectangle with melted butter and spread the walnut filling on top, leaving the far long edge of the dough uncovered by the filling.
6. Carefully and tightly roll the dough lengthwise. Pinch together the ends and transfer the prepared rolls to a piece of 12archment 12aP-er with the seams side down and wrap with cling wraP-,. Repeat with the other 2 dough pieces.
7. Let the rolls rise for 50-60 minutes. Meanwhile, preheat the oven to 350°F.
8. Once risen, bake the Slovak Kolache for 30- 40 minutes until golden. Transfer to a wire rack and cool completely before slicing. ENJOY!

APPETIZERS

BRUSCHETTA AL POMODORO
(CLASSIC TOMATO BRUSCHETTA)

INGREDIENTS

- 1 rustic Italian baguette or ciabatta, sliced into 1/2-inch rounds
- 4-5 ripe Roma tomatoes, deseeded and finely diced
- 1/4 cup extra-virgin olive oil, plus extra for drizzling
- 2 garlic cloves (1 halved, 1 minced)
- Fresh basil leaves, finely chopped
- Salt and freshly ground black pepper
- **Optional:** A splash of aged balsamic vinegar

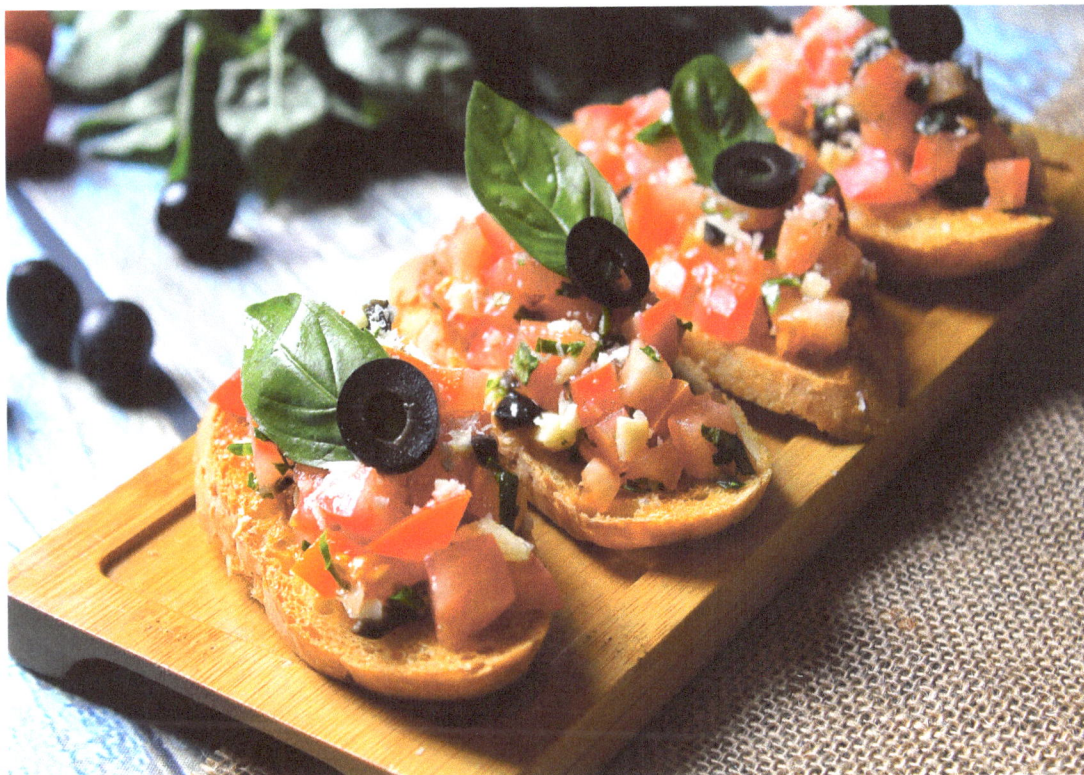

DIRECTIONS

STEP 1
PREPARE THE BREAD

Preheat oven to 400°F (200°C). Lay baguette slices on a baking sheet and lightly brush with olive oil. Toast for 8-10 minutes until golden and crisp, then rub each slice with the halved garlic clove.

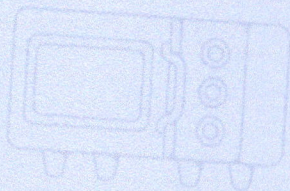

STEP 2
TOMATO MIXTURE

In a bowl, gently combine diced tomatoes, minced garlic, basil, 1/4 cup olive oil, salt, pepper, and balsamic if desired. Let sit for a few minutes to meld flavors.

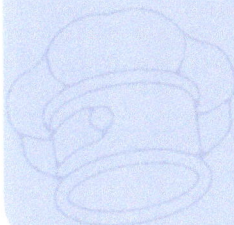

STEP 3
ASSEMBLE AND SERVE

Spoon the tomato mixture generously onto each toasted slice. Finish with a drizzle of olive oil for extra richness.

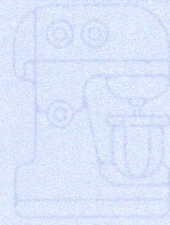

ARANCINI DI RISO
(CRISPY SICILIAN RICE BALLS)

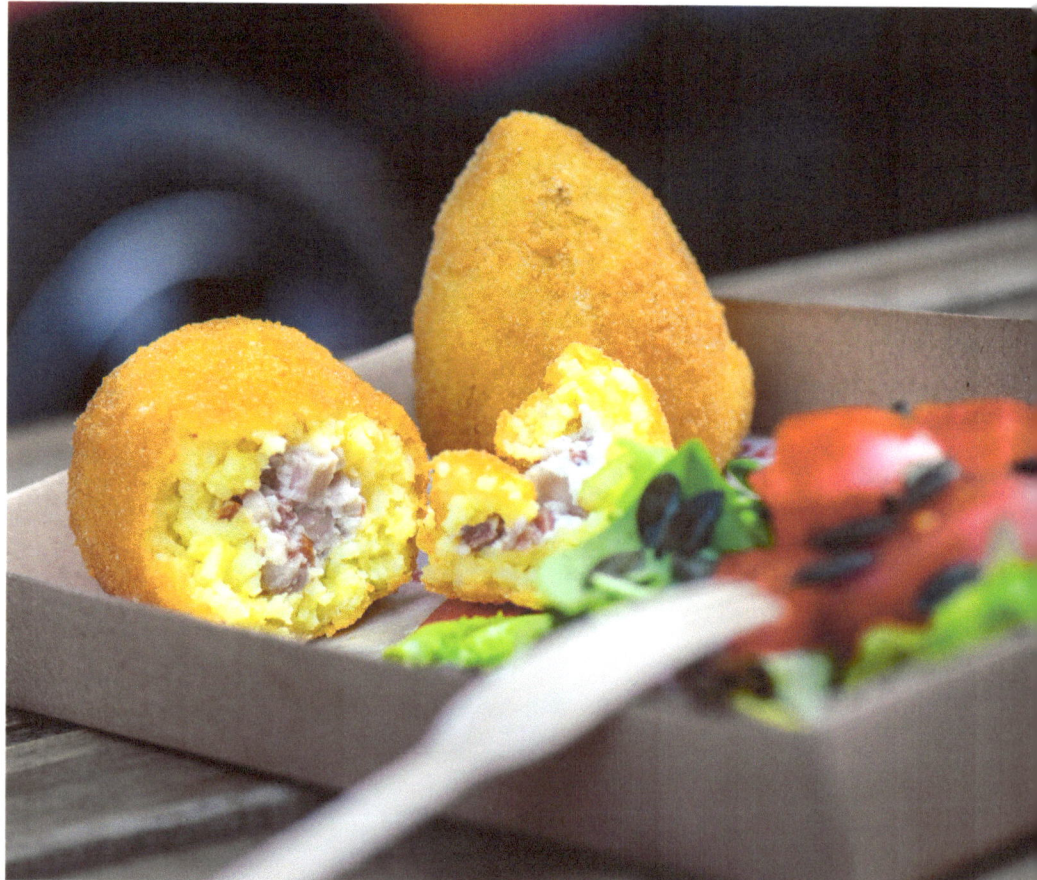

INGREDIENTS

- 2 cups cooked Arborio rice (cooled)
- 1/2 cup grated Parmesan cheese
- 1 large egg, beaten
- Small cubes of mozzarella
- 1 cup marinara sauce (for serving)
- 1/2 cup flour
- 2 eggs, beaten (for coating)
- 1 cup Italian breadcrumbs
- Vegetable oil for frying

DIRECTIONS

STEP 1
PREPARE RICE MIXTURE

In a large bowl, combine cooled rice, Parmesan, and the beaten egg until mixture is sticky enough to shape.

STEP 2
FORM ARANCINI

Take about 2 tablespoons of rice mixture, flatten in your palm, place a mozzarella cube in the center, and shape into a ball, ensuring mozzarella is fully covered.

STEP 3
BREADING

Coat each ball in flour, dip in beaten eggs, and roll in breadcrumbs.

STEP 4
BREADING

Heat oil to 350°F (175°C) and fry in batches until golden brown. Drain on paper towels and serve hot with marinara.

CROSTINI WITH RICOTTA AND HONEY

- 1 baguette, sliced and lightly toasted
- 1 cup high-quality ricotta cheese, drained
- Honey for drizzling
- Fresh thyme leaves for garnish
- Flaky sea salt and freshly ground black pepper

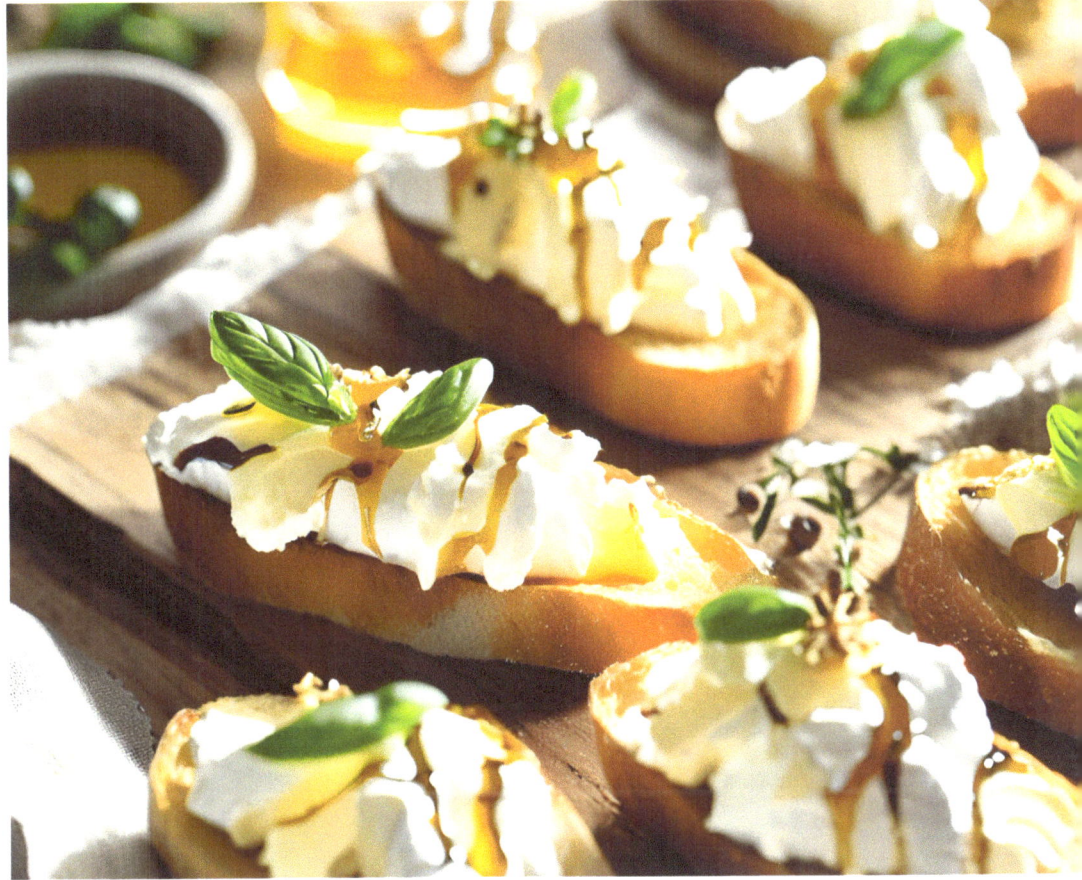

DIRECTIONS

STEP 1
TOAST BREAD

Toast baguette slices until golden, either in a skillet or under the broiler.

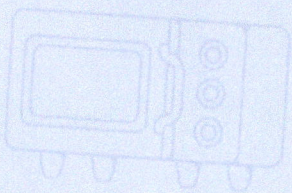

STEP 2
SPREAD AND GARNISH

Spoon ricotta onto each toast, drizzle with honey, and sprinkle with fresh thyme.

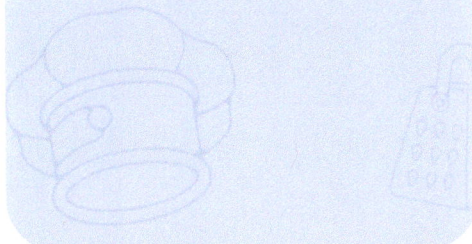

STEP 3
FINISH AND SERVE

Add a pinch of sea salt and black pepper. Serve warm or at room temperature.

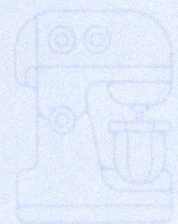

CAPRESE SKEWERS

- 1 pint grape tomatoes
- 1 container mini mozzarella balls (bocconcini)
- Fresh basil leaves (See Fresh Mozzarella Recipe)
- Balsamic glaze for drizzling
- Sea salt and cracked black pepper

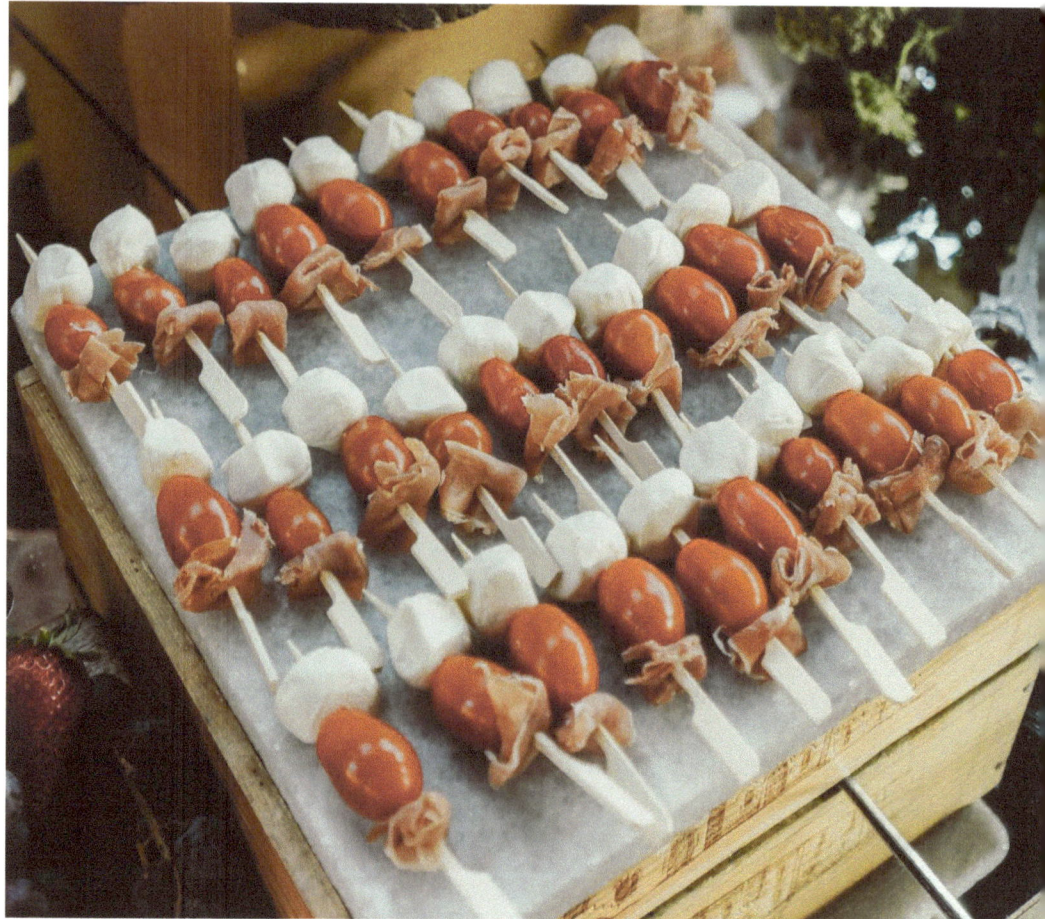

DIRECTIONS

STEP 1
ASSEMBLE SKEWERS

On small skewers, alternate a cherry tomato, basil leaf, and mozzarella ball.

STEP 2
PLATE AND DRIZZLE

Arrange on a platter and drizzle with balsamic glaze. Season with a light sprinkling of salt and pepper just before serving.

PROSCIUTTO-WRAPPED MELON

- 1 ripe cantaloupe, peeled and sliced into wedges
- 12-15 slices of prosciutto
- Fresh mint or basil leaves for garnish

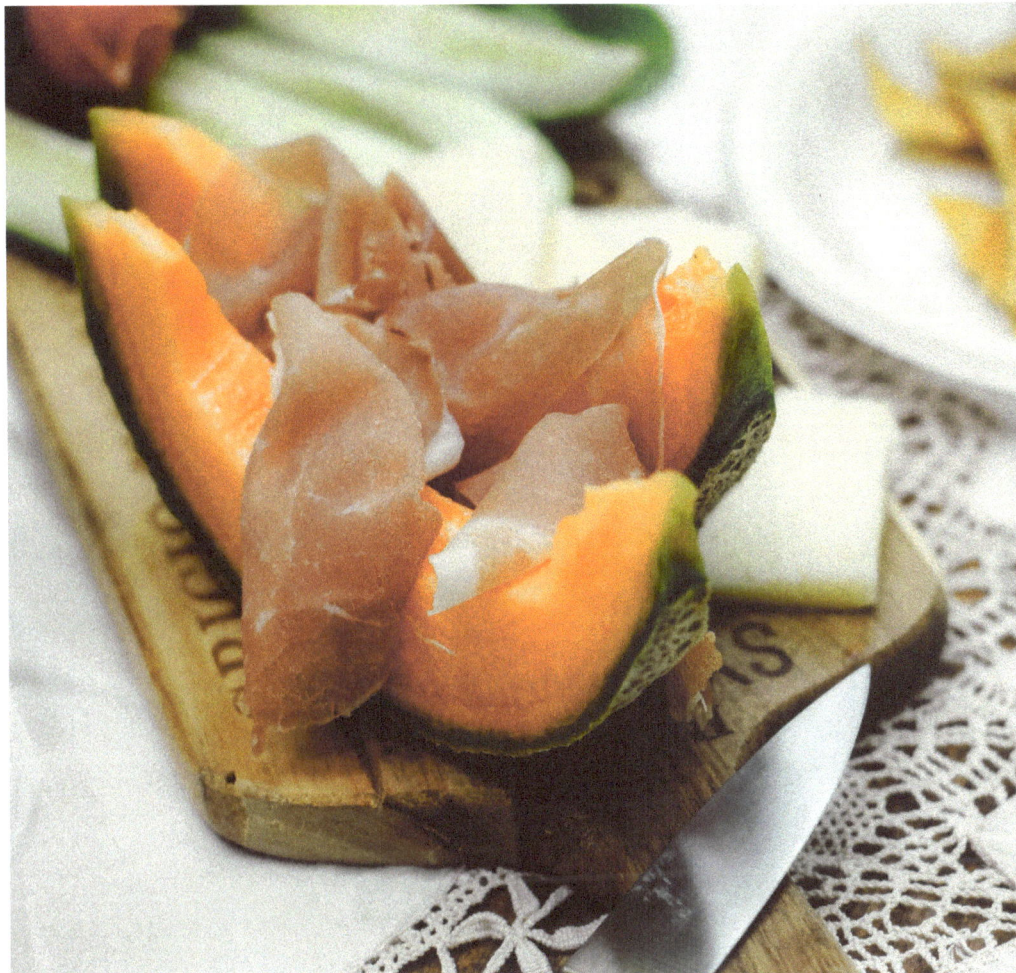

DIRECTIONS

STEP 1
WRAP MELON

Wrap each melon slice in a prosciutto slice, securing it firmly.

STEP 2
GARNISH AND SERVE

Arrange on a platter with basil or mint leaves, which add freshness to balance the sweetness and saltiness.

KERRY'S STUFFED MUSHROOMS WITH ITALIAN SAUSAGE

INGREDIENTS

- 1 lb large button mushrooms, stems removed and saved
- 1/2 lb Italian sausage
- 1/4 cup grated Parmesan cheese
- 1/4 cup breadcrumbs
- 1 tbsp fresh parsley, chopped
- 1 clove garlic, minced
- Olive oil for drizzling

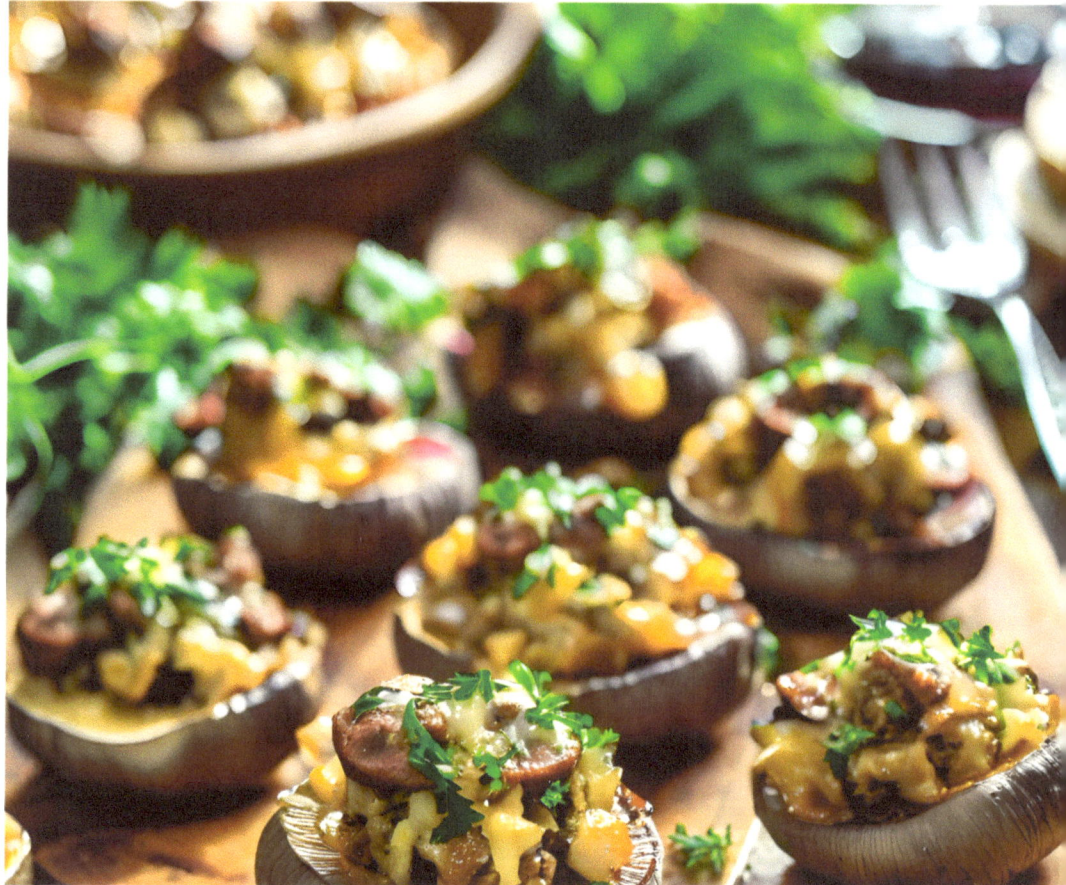

DIRECTIONS

STEP 1
COOK SAUSAGE FILLING

In a skillet, brown sausage, breaking it up as it cooks. Add chopped mushroom stems, parsley, garlic, breadcrumbs, and Parmesan, stirring to combine.

STEP 2
STUFF AND BAKE

Fill each mushroom cap with the sausage mixture, place on a baking sheet, and drizzle with olive oil. Bake at 375°F (190°C) for 15-20 minutes until golden and bubbling.

ZUCCHINI FRITTATA BITES

INGREDIENTS

- 3 large eggs, lightly beaten
- 1/2 cup zucchini, thinly sliced
- 1/4 cup grated Parmesan cheese
- 1/4 cup fresh parsley, chopped
- Salt and pepper to taste
- Olive oil for cooking

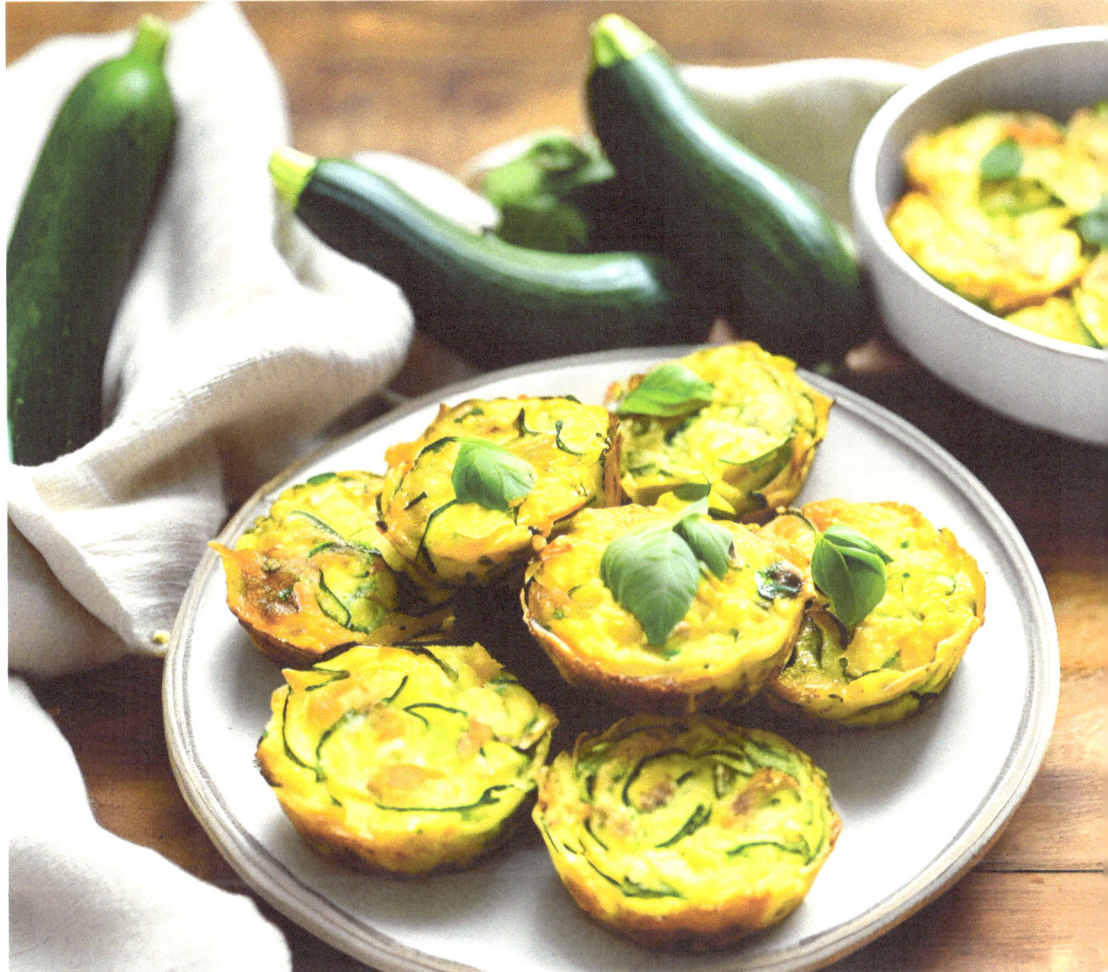

DIRECTIONS

STEP 1
SAUTÉ ZUCCHINI

In a skillet over medium heat, cook zucchini with a touch of olive oil until softened.

STEP 2
COOK FRITTATA

Add eggs, Parmesan, parsley, salt, and pepper, and cook gently until set. Flip if needed, cut into squares, and serve.

EGGPLANT ROLLATINI

INGREDIENTS

- 1 large eggplant, peeled, sliced lengthwise into thin strips
- 1 cup ricotta cheese
- 1/4 cup Parmesan cheese
- 1 cup marinara sauce
- Fresh basil leaves, chopped
- 2 whole eggs beaten
- Half cup flour, season with salt and pepper

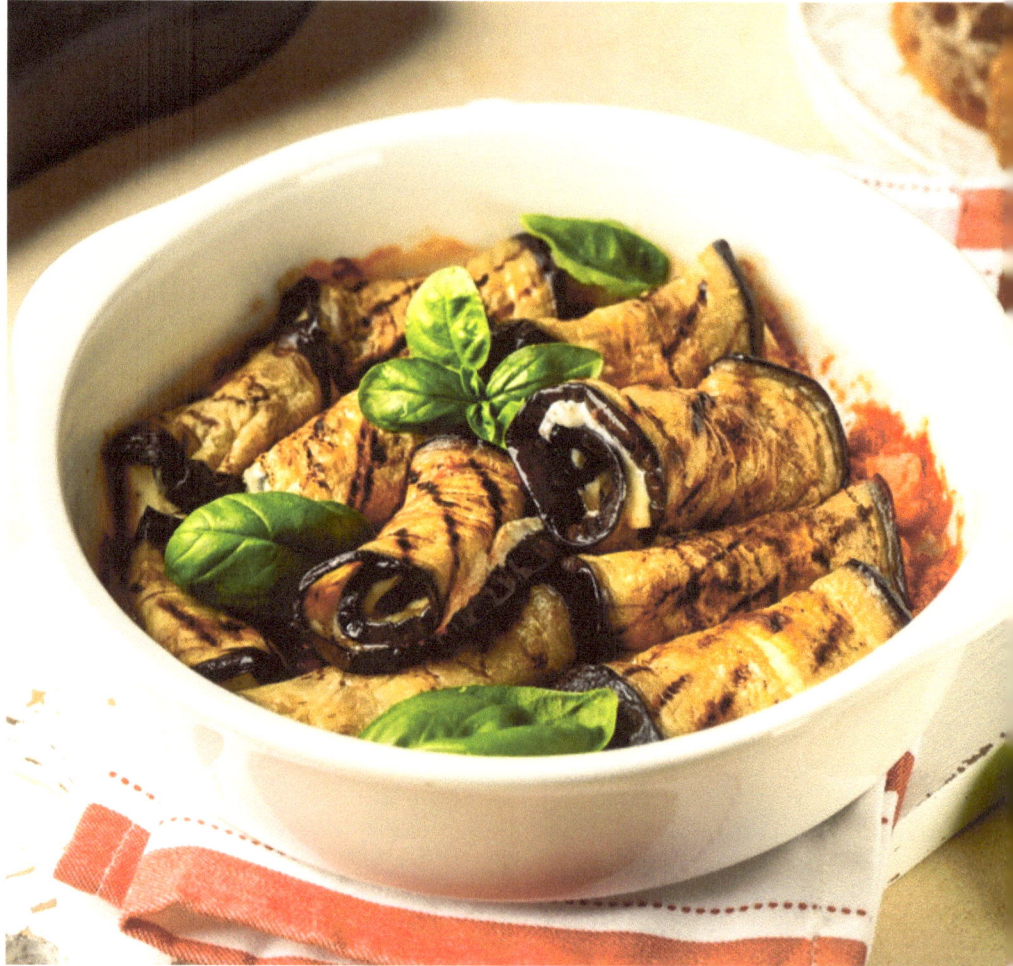

DIRECTIONS

STEP 1
DREDGE

Eggplant in flour, then egg, and sauté in a pan with hot oil until golden brown-remove and reserve.

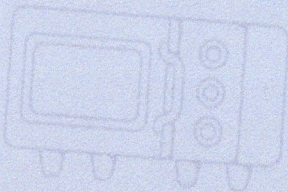

STEP 2
FILL AND ROLL

Place a spoonful of ricotta and Parmesan mixture on each slice, roll up, and place in a baking dish with marinara sauce.

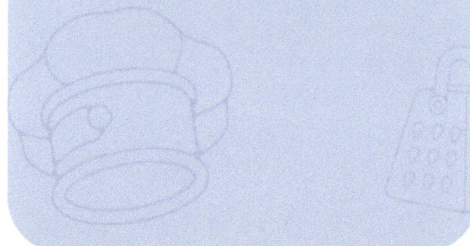

STEP 3
BAKE AND SERVE

Top with remaining sauce and bake until bubbly, then garnish with basil.

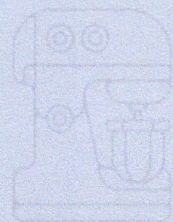

ANTIPASTO PLATTER

INGREDIENTS

- Italian cured meats (prosciutto, salami, capicola)
- Italian cheeses (Provolone, Parmigiano-Reggiano)
- Marinated olives, roasted red peppers, artichoke hearts
- Grissini (Italian breadsticks)

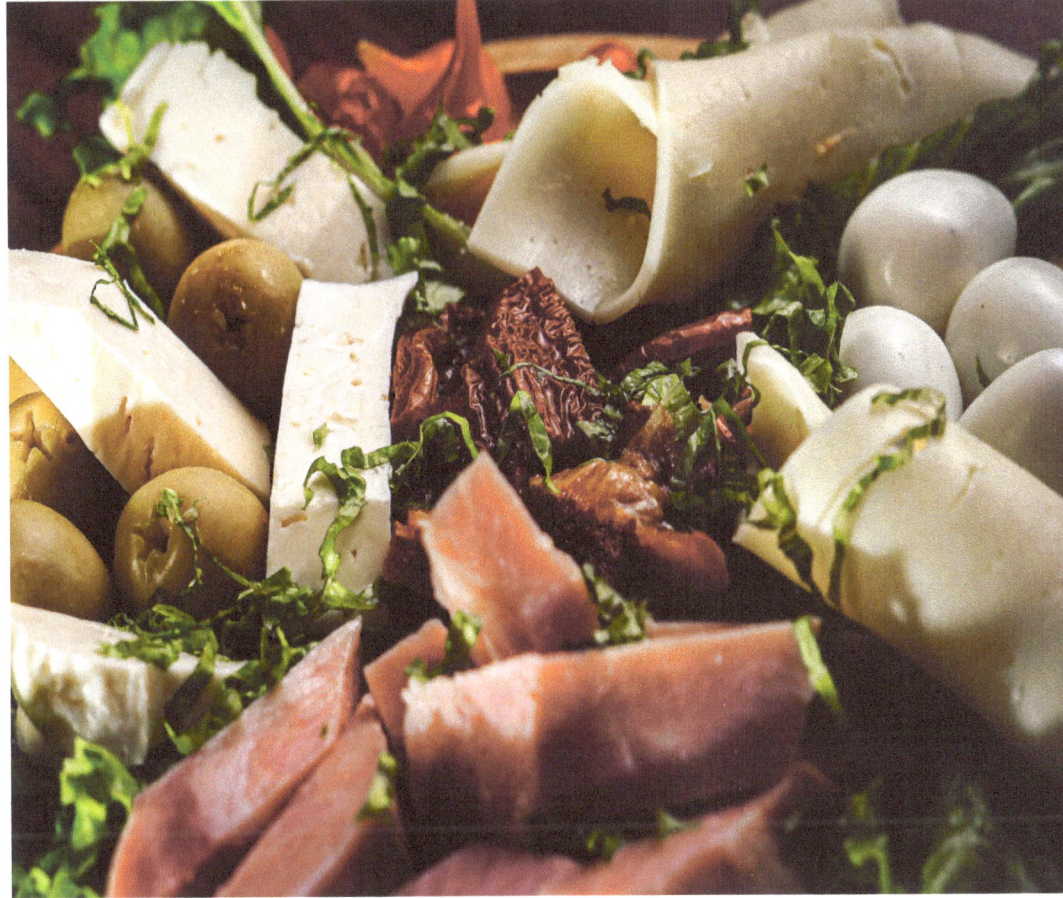

DIRECTIONS

STEP 1
ASSEMBLE PLATTER

Arrange each item in its own section on a large serving board.

STEP 2
GARNISH AND SERVE

Add fresh herbs like rosemary or basil for a visual pop and serve with breadsticks.

POLENTA BITES WITH MUSHROOM RAGU

INGREDIENTS

- 1 cup polenta
- 4 cups chicken or vegetable broth
- 1/4 cup Parmesan cheese
- 1/4 cup mushrooms, finely diced
- 1 clove garlic, minced
- Olive oil for cooking

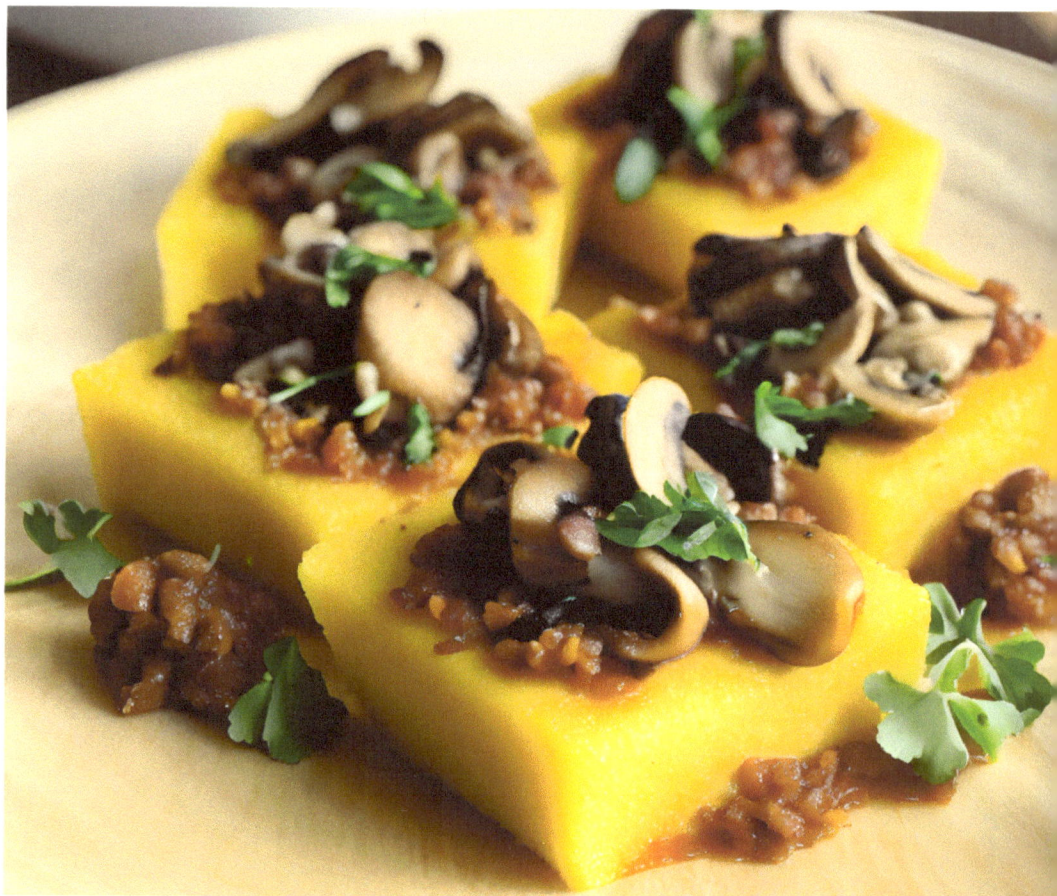

DIRECTIONS

STEP 1
COOK POLENTA

Simmer broth, then whisk in polenta and cook until thickened. Stir in Parmesan, spread onto a sheet to cool, and cut into squares.

STEP 2
PREPARE MUSHROOM RAGU

Sauté mushrooms and garlic in olive oil. Top each polenta square with the mushroom ragu and serve warm.

FRITTELLE DI ZUCCHINE (ZUCCHINI FRITTERS)

INGREDIENTS

- 2 medium zucchinis, grated
- 1/4 cup Parmesan cheese, grated
- 1/2 cup all-purpose flour
- 1 egg, beaten
- Salt and black pepper
- Olive oil for frying
- **Optional:** fresh herbs (parsley, basil), chopped

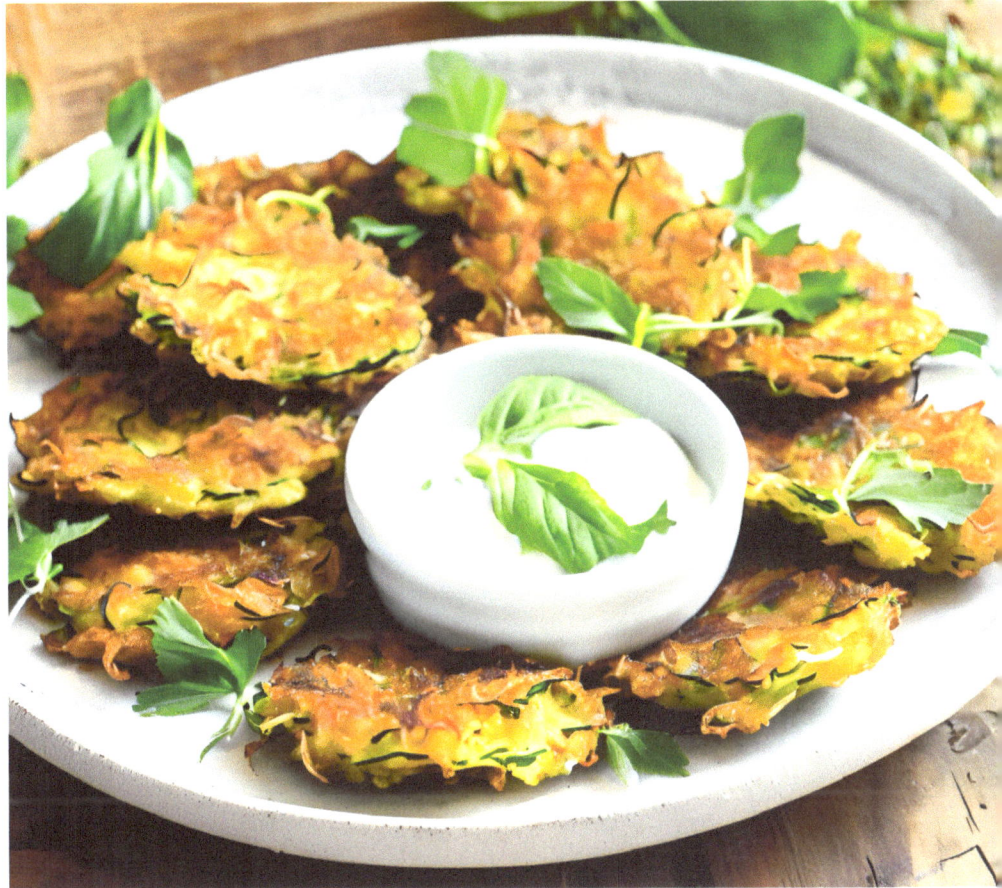

DIRECTIONS

STEP 1
PREP ZUCCHINI

Place grated zucchini in a bowl with a pinch of salt, let it sit for 10 minutes, then squeeze out any excess liquid.

STEP 2
MAKE BATTER

Combine zucchini, flour, Parmesan, egg, and herbs. Season with salt and pepper.

STEP 3
FRY FRITTERS

Heat a thin layer of olive oil in a skillet over medium heat. Drop spoonfuls of the batter, flatten slightly, and cook until golden, about 3-4 minutes per side. Drain on paper towels.

CAPONATA
(SICILIAN EGGPLANT SALAD)

INGREDIENTS

- 2 medium eggplants, diced
- 1/4 cup olive oil
- 1 onion, chopped
- 2 stalks celery, chopped
- 1/4 cup green olives, pitted and chopped
- 2 tbsp capers
- 1/4 cup red wine vinegar
- 2 tbsp sugar
- 1/4 cup tomato paste

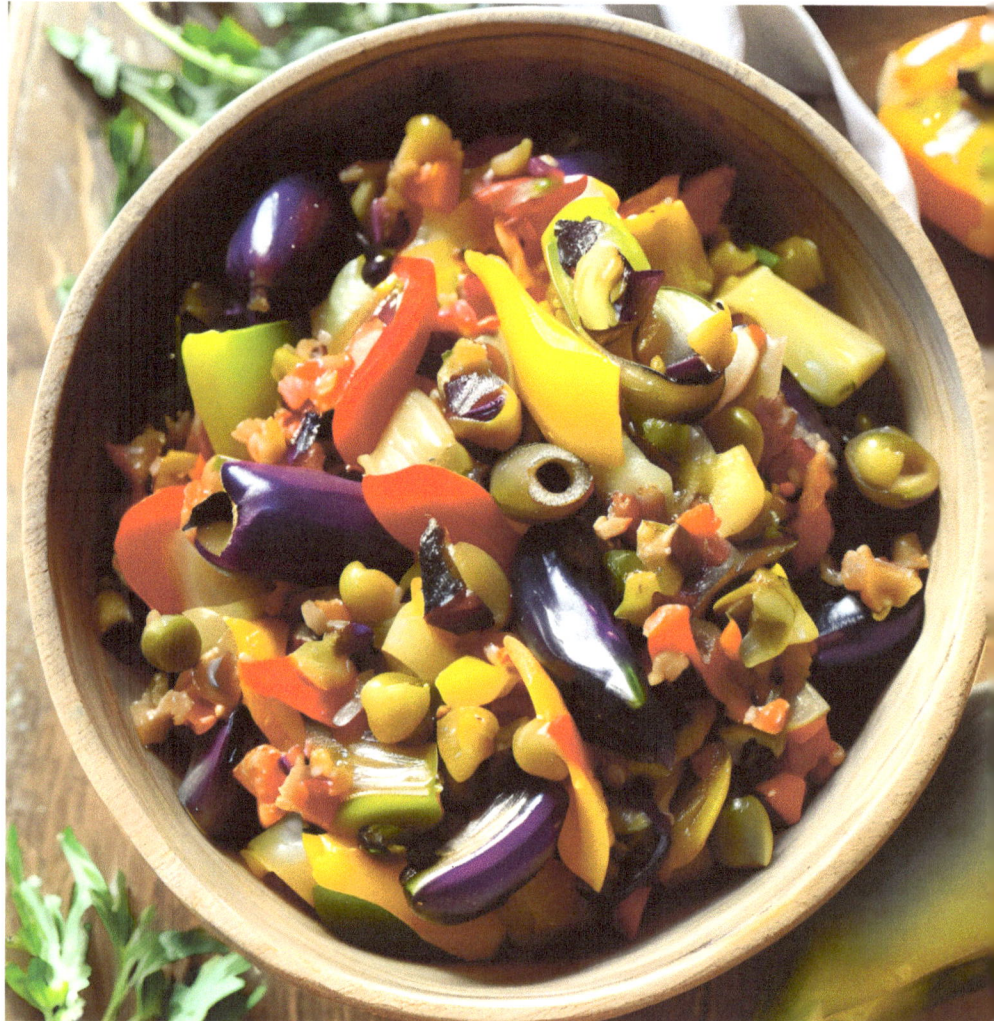

DIRECTIONS

STEP 1
COOK EGGPLANT

Heat olive oil in a large skillet, add eggplant, and cook until tender and browned. Set aside.

STEP 2
SAUTÉ VEGETABLES

In the same skillet, cook onion and celery until soft. Add olives, capers, tomato paste, vinegar, and sugar. Simmer for 10-15 minutes until thickened, then fold in the eggplant. Serve warm or at room temperature.

MOZZARELLA IN CARROZZA
(FRIED MOZZARELLA SANDWICHES)

INGREDIENTS

- 8 slices of white bread
- 8 oz fresh mozzarella, sliced
- 2 eggs, beaten
- 1 cup milk
- 1 cup Italian breadcrumbs
- Olive oil for frying

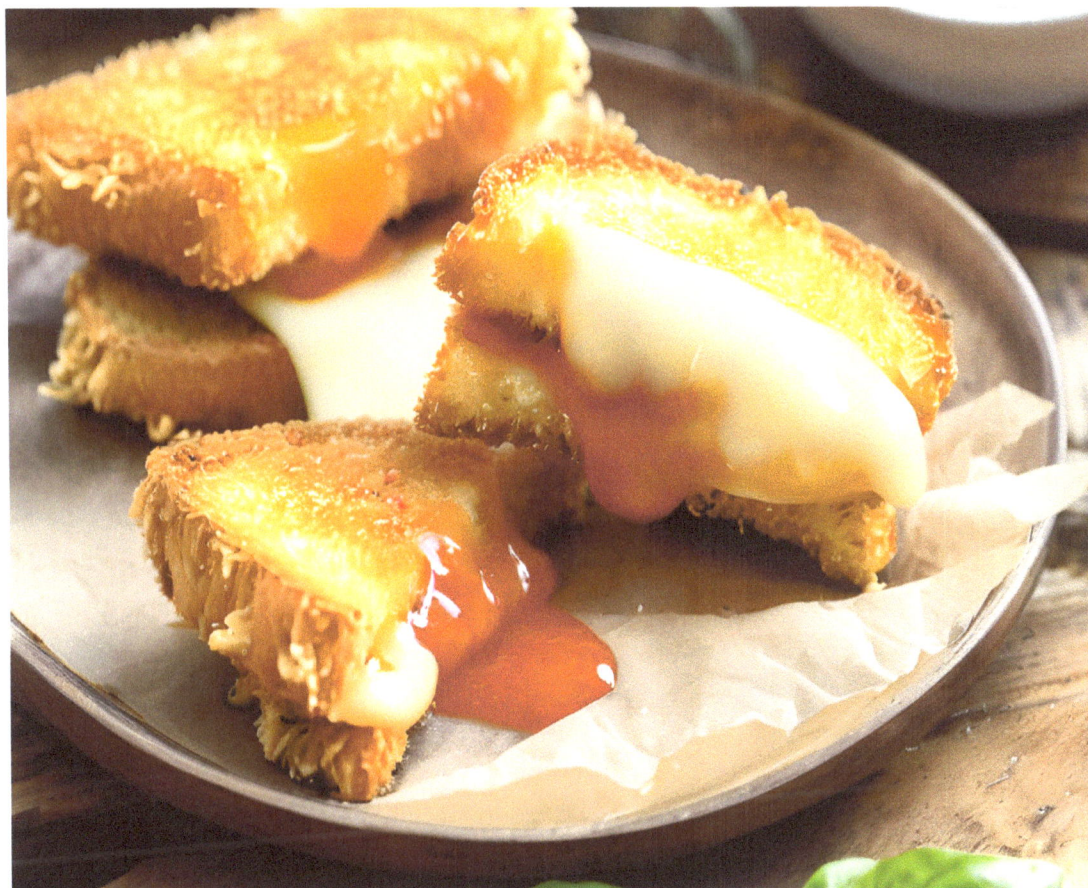

DIRECTIONS

STEP 1
ASSEMBLE SANDWICHES

Place mozzarella between two slices of bread, press firmly, and trim edges.

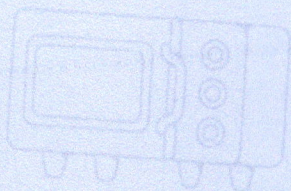

STEP 2
BREAD THE SANDWICHES

Dip each sandwich in milk, then coat in beaten egg, and finally in breadcrumbs.

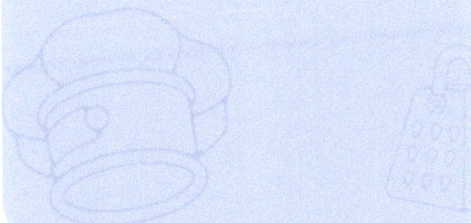

STEP 3
FRY

Heat oil in a skillet, fry sandwiches until golden and crispy on both sides. Drain and slice into triangles.

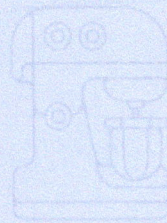

INSALATA DI POLPO
(OCTOPUS SALAD)

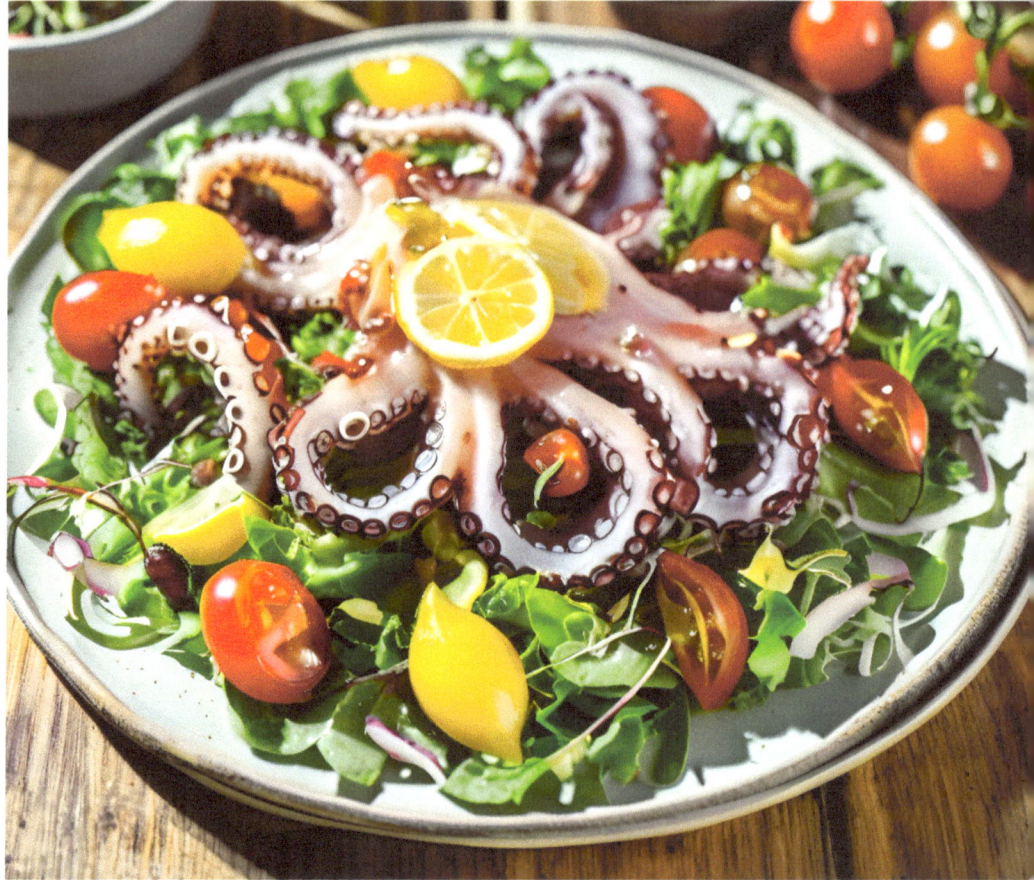

INGREDIENTS

- 1 lb octopus, cleaned
- 1 lemon, sliced
- 1 bay leaf
- 1/4 cup extra-virgin olive oil
- 1/2 cup cherry tomatoes, halved
- Fresh parsley, chopped
- Salt and pepper

DIRECTIONS

STEP 1
COOK OCTOPUS

Bring a pot of water with lemon and bay leaf to a boil, then simmer octopus until tender, about 45 minutes. Cool and slice.

STEP 2
ASSEMBLE SALAD

Toss octopus, tomatoes, parsley, olive oil, salt, and pepper in a bowl. Chill before serving.

BURRATA WITH ROASTED TOMATOES AND BASIL OIL

INGREDIENTS

- 1 pint cherry tomatoes
- 1 tbsp olive oil
- Salt and pepper
- 8 oz burrata cheese
- 1/4 cup basil leaves, finely chopped
- Extra-virgin olive oil for drizzling

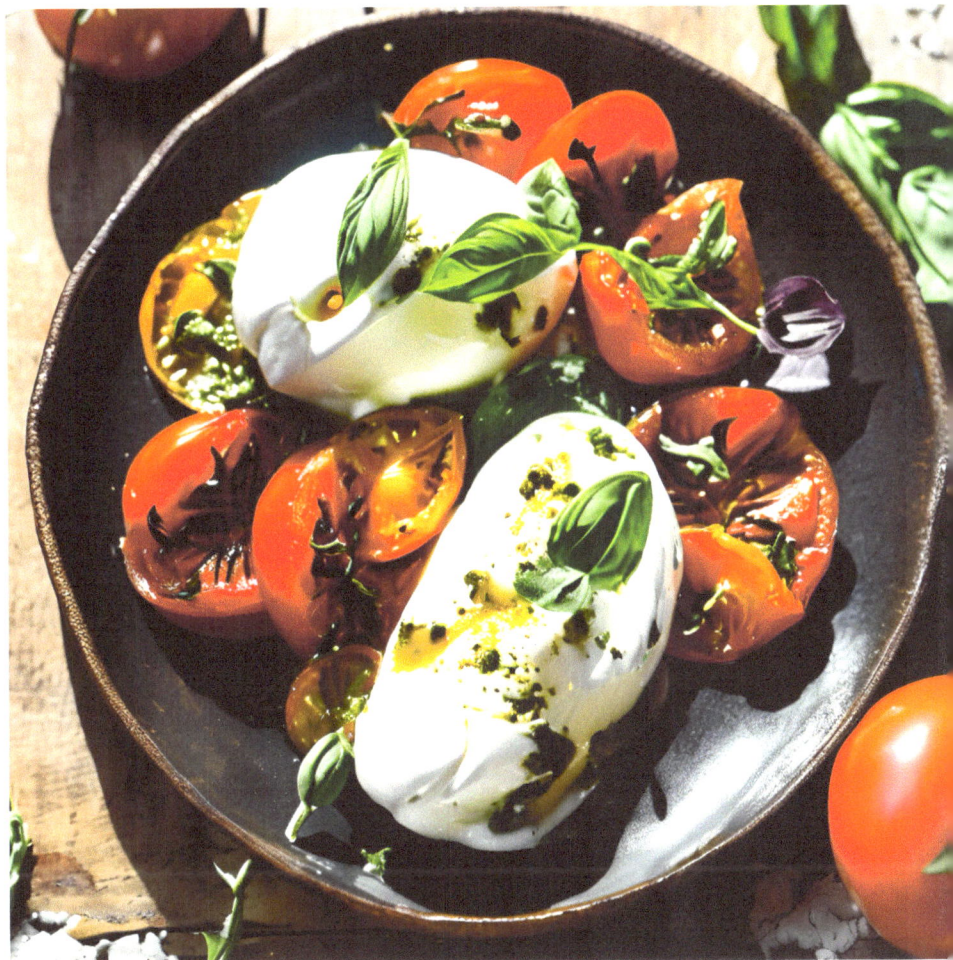

DIRECTIONS

STEP 1
ROAST TOMATOES

Preheat oven to 400°F. Toss tomatoes with olive oil, salt, and pepper, and roast for 15 minutes.

STEP 2
ASSEMBLE

Place burrata on a serving plate, scatter roasted tomatoes, drizzle with basil oil, and garnish with basil.

CANNELLINI BEAN DIP WITH ROSEMARY AND GARLIC

INGREDIENTS

- 1 can cannellini beans, drained and rinsed
- 1 garlic clove, minced
- 2 tbsp fresh rosemary, chopped
- 1/4 cup olive oil
- Salt and pepper
- Red pepper flakes (optional)

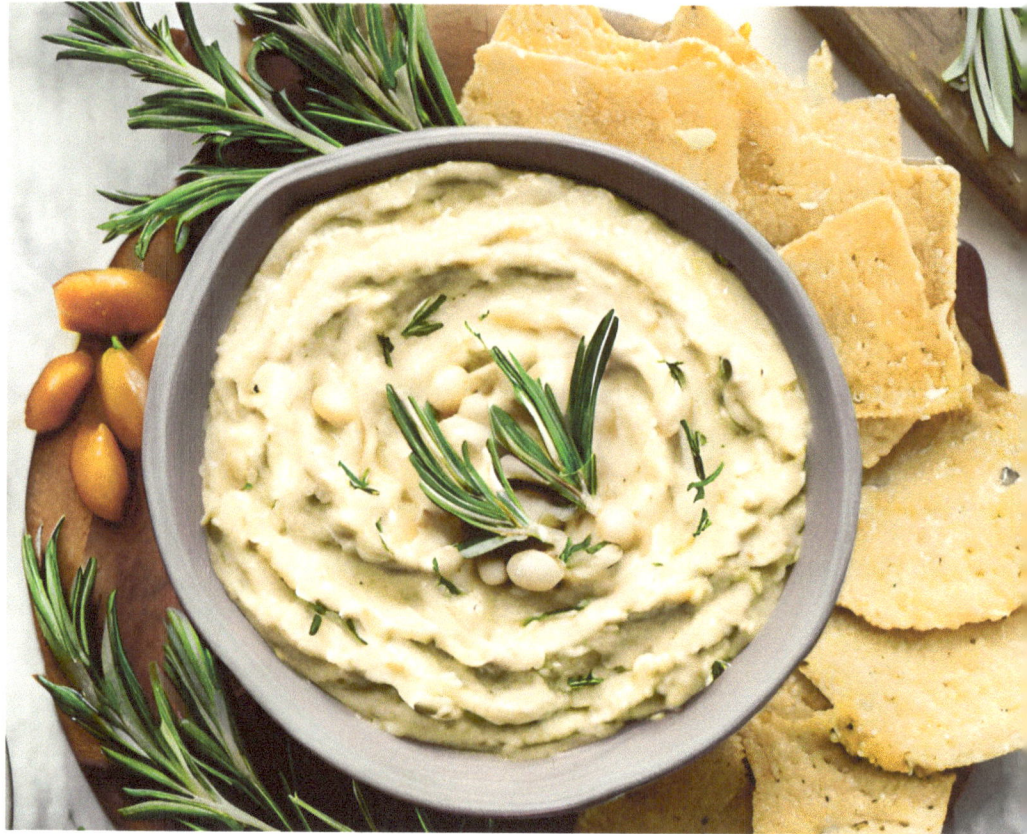

DIRECTIONS

STEP 1
BLEND DIP

Combine beans, garlic, rosemary, olive oil, salt, and pepper in a food processor. Blend until smooth.

STEP 2
SERVE

Spoon into a bowl, drizzle with extra olive oil, and sprinkle with red pepper flakes.

STUFFED CALAMARI

INGREDIENTS

- 1 lb squid tubes, cleaned
- 1/2 cup breadcrumbs
- 1/4 cup Parmesan, grated
- 2 tbsp fresh parsley, chopped
- 2 cloves garlic, minced
- 1/4 cup olive oil
- 1 lemon, for zest and juice

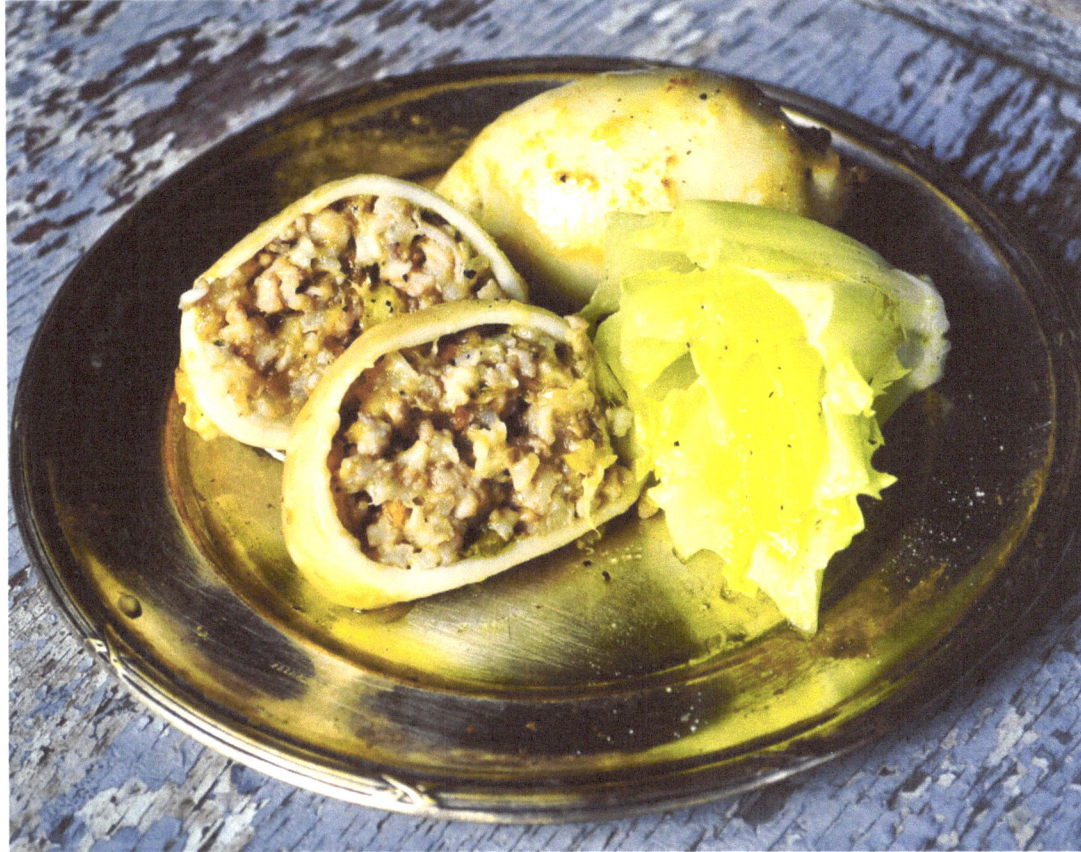

DIRECTIONS

STEP 1
MAKE FILLING

Mix breadcrumbs, Parmesan, parsley, garlic, lemon zest, and half the olive oil.

STEP 2
STUFF CALAMARI

Fill each squid tube with the mixture, securing the ends with toothpicks.

STEP 3
COOK

Sear in a hot skillet with remaining oil for 4-5 minutes per side, until squid is opaque and tender.

PROSCIUTTO AND FIG CROSTINI

- 1 baguette, sliced and toasted
- 1/2 cup ricotta cheese
- 6 fresh figs, sliced
- 8 slices prosciutto
- Honey, for drizzling
- Fresh thyme leaves, for garnish

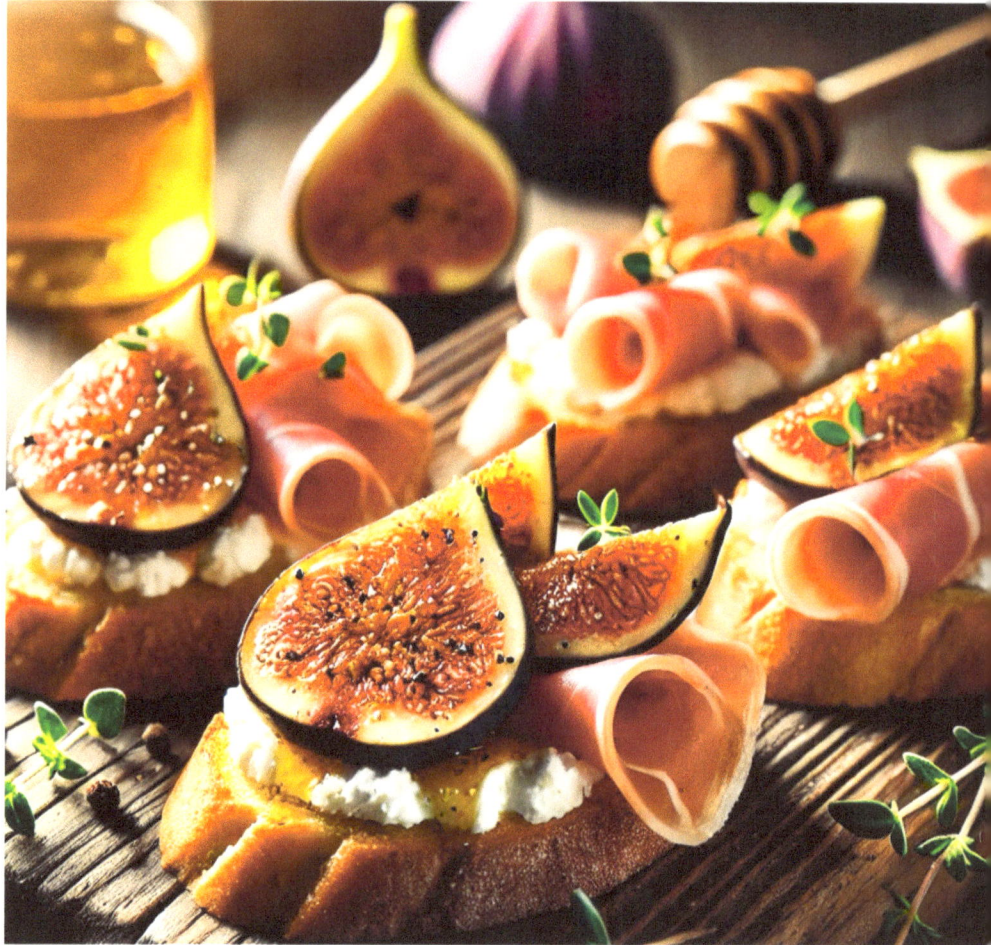

DIRECTIONS

STEP 1
ASSEMBLE CROSTINI

Spread ricotta on each toast, top with fig slices and prosciutto.

STEP 2
GARNISH AND SERVE

Drizzle with honey and sprinkle with thyme.

MARINATED ARTICHOKES AND OLIVES

INGREDIENTS

- 1 cup artichoke hearts, halved
- 1 cup mixed olives
- 1/4 cup olive oil
- 1/4 cup white wine vinegar
- 1 clove garlic, minced
- Fresh rosemary, thyme, and parsley

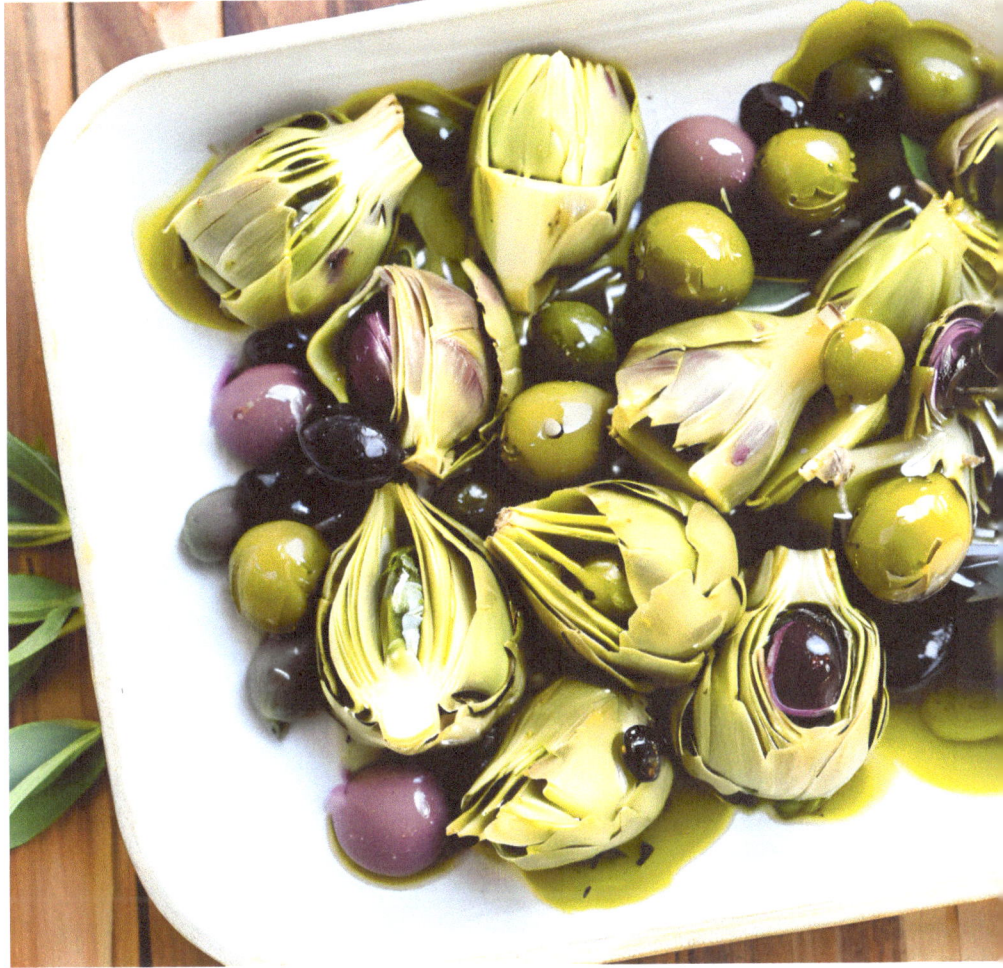

DIRECTIONS

STEP 1
MAKE MARINADE

Whisk together olive oil, vinegar, garlic, and herbs.

STEP 2
COMBINE

Toss artichokes and olives in the marinade, cover, and refrigerate for at least 1 hour.

GORGONZOLA-STUFFED DATES WRAPPED IN PANCETTA

INGREDIENTS

- 12 large Medjool dates, pitted
- 1/4 cup Gorgonzola cheese
- 12 slices pancetta

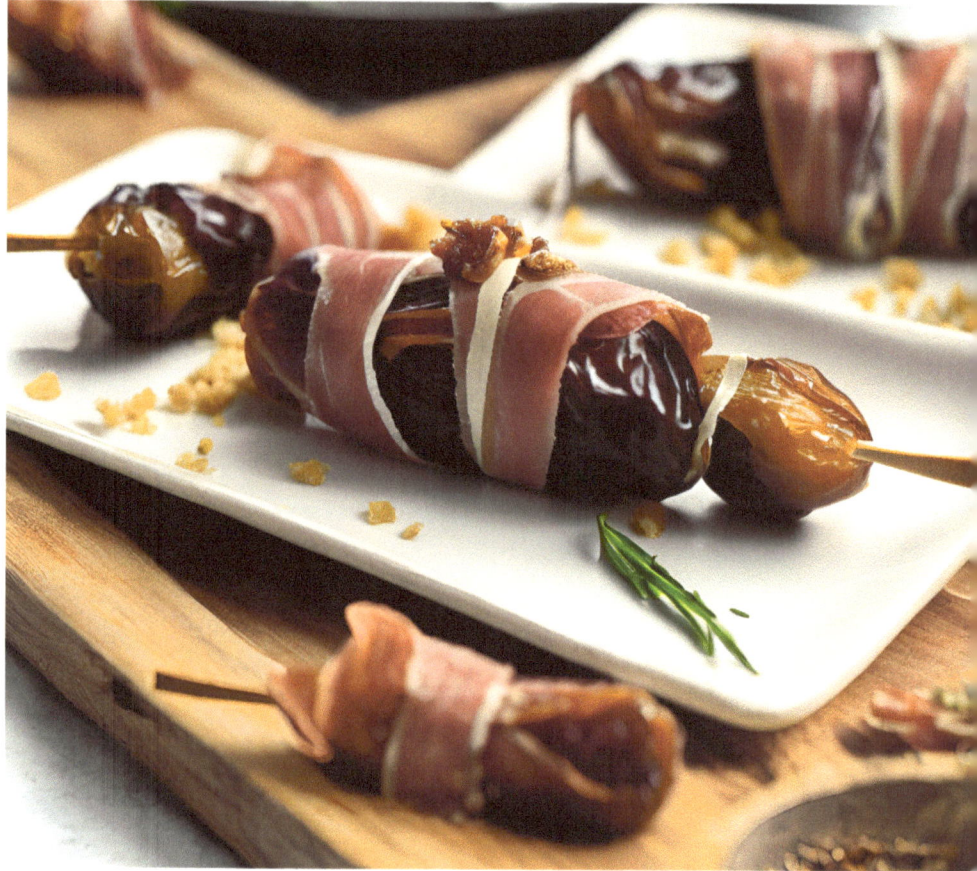

DIRECTIONS

STEP 1
FILL DATES

Stuff each date with Gorgonzola.

STEP 2
WRAP IN PANCETTA

Wrap each date in pancetta and secure with a toothpick.

STEP 3
BAKE AND SERVE

Place on a baking sheet and bake at 375°F for 10-12 minutes until pancetta is crispy. Serve warm.

SALADS

ITALIAN PANZANELLA SALAD

INGREDIENTS

- 4 cups stale or toasted bread cubes
- 1 lb ripe tomatoes, chopped
- 1 cucumber, thinly sliced
- 1 red bell pepper, chopped
- 1/2 red onion, thinly sliced
- 1/4 cup fresh basil leaves, torn
- 1/4 cup olive oil
- 2 tbsp red wine vinegar
- Salt and black pepper to taste

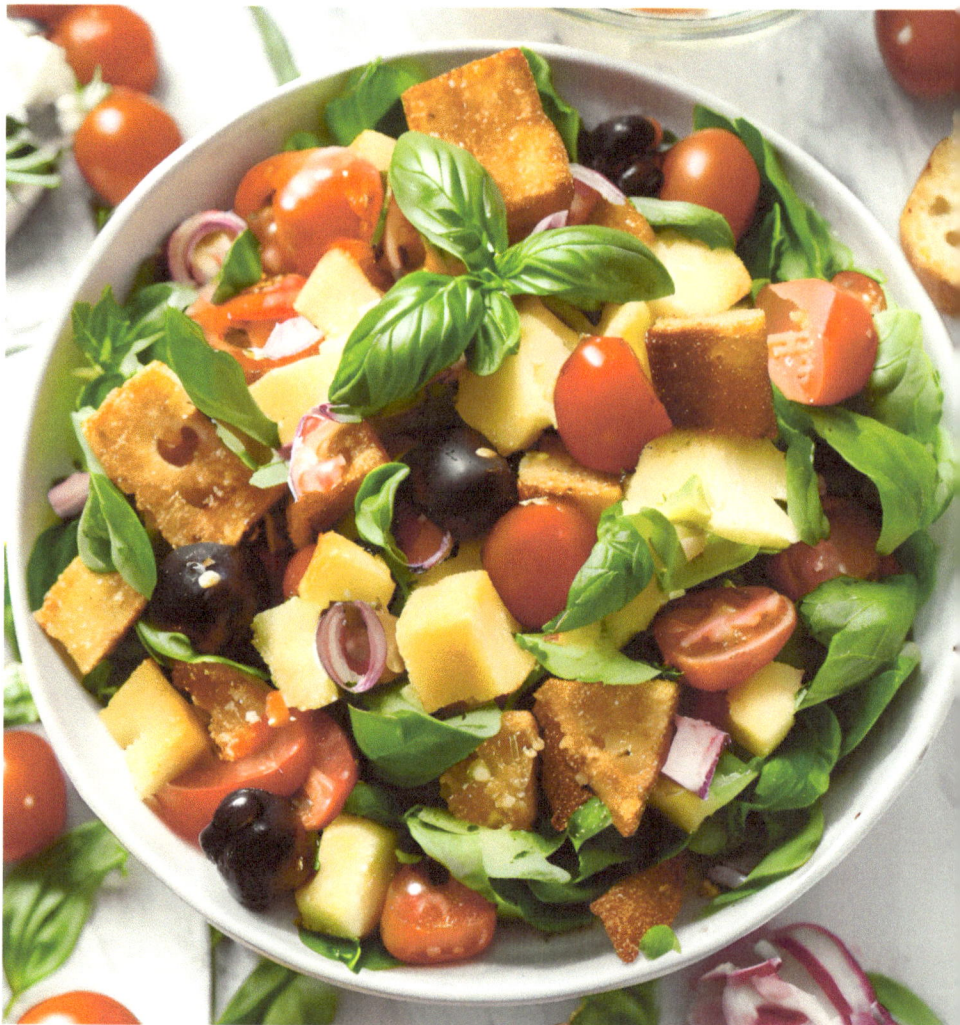

DIRECTIONS

STEP 1
TOAST THE BREAD

Cut the bread into 1-inch cubes. If using fresh bread, toast in a preheated oven at 350°F (175°C) for 10 minutes until golden and crispy. This helps prevent sogginess when dressing the salad.

STEP 2
PREPARE THE VEGETABLES

Dice the tomatoes and slice the cucumber thinly. Chop the red bell pepper into small cubes, and thinly slice the red onion. Add all vegetables to a large mixing bowl.

STEP 3
MAKE THE DRESSING

In a small bowl, whisk together the olive oil, red wine vinegar, salt, and pepper. Adjust the seasoning as needed.

STEP 4
ASSEMBLE THE SALAD

Add the toasted bread cubes to the bowl with the vegetables. Pour the dressing over and gently toss everything to combine.

STEP 5
ADD BASIL

Tear the basil leaves by hand and sprinkle them over the salad. Let it sit for 10-15 minutes to allow the flavors to blend.

STEP 6
SERVE

Toss lightly once more and serve as a refreshing, rustic appetizer.

CAPRESE SALAD WITH BALSAMIC REDUCTION

INGREDIENTS

- 2 large ripe tomatoes, sliced
- 8 oz fresh mozzarella, sliced (See fresh mozzarella recipe)
- Fresh basil leaves
- 1/4 cup balsamic vinegar
- 2 tbsp extra-virgin olive oil
- Salt and black pepper to taste

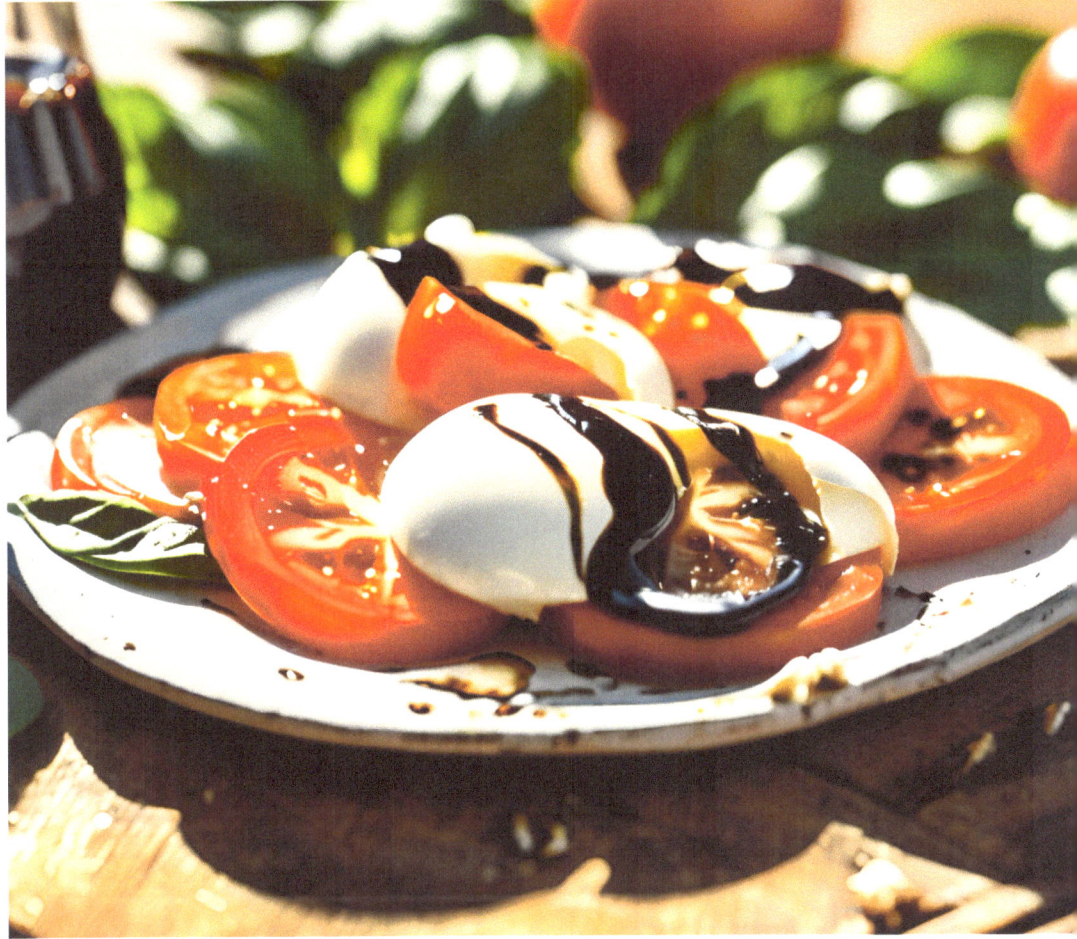

DIRECTIONS

STEP 1
PREPARE THE BALSAMIC REDUCTION

Pour balsamic vinegar into a small saucepan and heat over medium heat. Simmer for about 5-7 minutes, stirring occasionally, until it thickens into a syrup. Set aside to cool.

STEP 2
ASSEMBLE THE SALAD

On a large serving plate, alternate slices of tomato, mozzarella, and basil leaves in a circular or linear arrangement.

STEP 3
DRIZZLE WITH OIL AND VINEGAR

Lightly drizzle the olive oil and reduced balsamic over the salad. Season with salt and pepper.

STEP 4
SERVE IMMEDIATELY

For the freshest taste, serve immediately, allowing guests to enjoy the creamy mozzarella with tangy tomatoes and aromatic basil.

ITALIAN FARRO SALAD

INGREDIENTS

- 1 cup farro, rinsed and drained
- 1 pint cherry tomatoes, halved
- 1/2 cup Kalamata olives, pitted and sliced
- 1/4 cup red onion, finely diced
- 1 cucumber, diced
- 1/4 cup fresh parsley, chopped
- 1/4 cup fresh basil, chopped
- 1/4 cup crumbled feta cheese
- 3 tbsp olive oil
- 2 tbsp red wine vinegar
- Salt and black pepper to taste

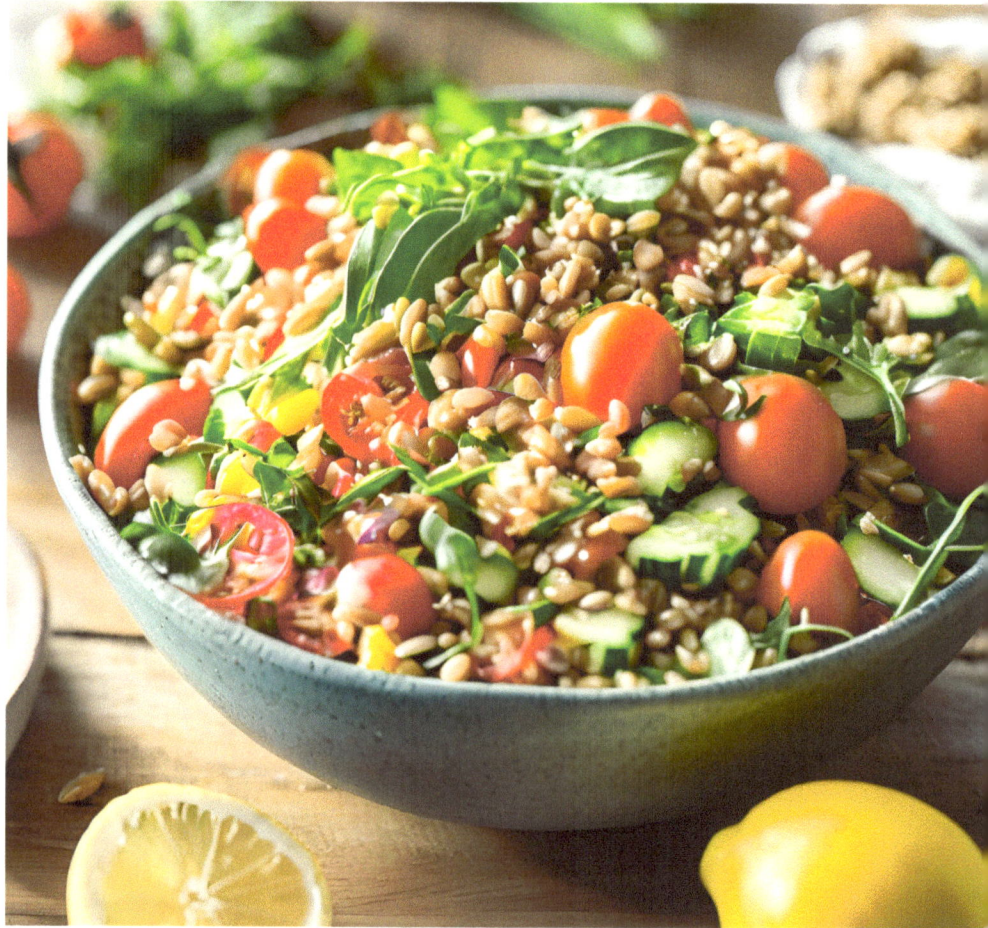

DIRECTIONS

STEP 1
COOK THE FARRO

In a medium pot, add the farro with 3 cups of water. Bring to a boil, then reduce heat and simmer for about 20-25 minutes until tender. Drain any excess water and allow farro to cool slightly.

STEP 2
CHOP VEGETABLES AND HERBS

While the farro is cooking, halve the cherry tomatoes, slice the olives, dice the onion and cucumber, and chop the parsley and basil.

STEP 3
MAKE THE DRESSING

In a small bowl, whisk together olive oil, red wine vinegar, salt, and pepper.

STEP 4
COMBINE INGREDIENTS

In a large bowl, mix the cooled farro with tomatoes, olives, onion, cucumber, parsley, and basil. Add the feta cheese.

STEP 5
DRESS AND SERVE

Pour the dressing over the salad and toss gently to combine. Serve immediately or chill in the refrigerator for a more refreshing taste.

ITALIAN CHOPPED ANTIPASTO SALAD

INGREDIENTS

- 1 head romaine lettuce, chopped
- 1/2 cup cherry tomatoes, halved
- 1/2 cup artichoke hearts, drained and chopped
- 1/4 cup black olives, sliced
- 1/4 cup green olives, sliced
- 1/4 cup roasted red peppers, diced
- 1/4 cup salami slices, chopped
- 1/4 cup provolone cheese, cubed
- 1/4 cup red onion, diced
- 3 tbsp red wine vinegar
- 1/4 cup olive oil
- Salt and pepper to taste

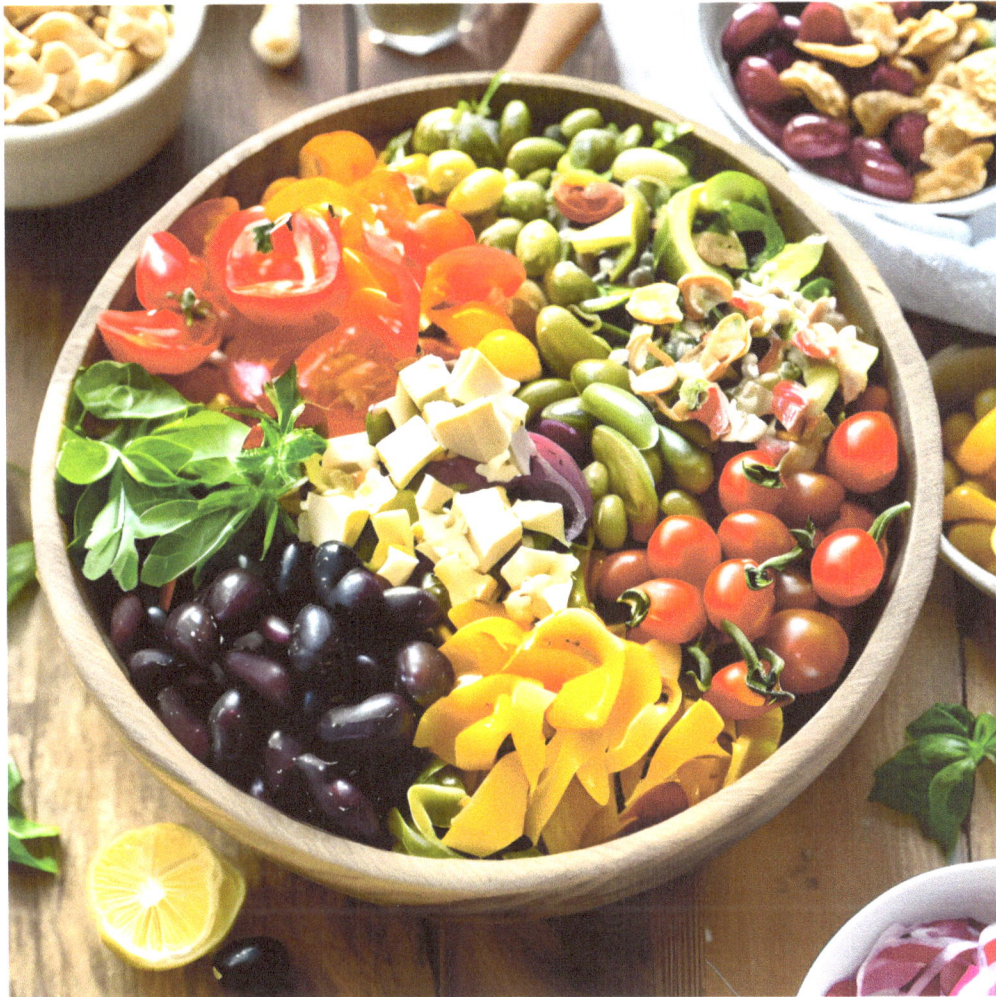

DIRECTIONS

STEP 1
PREPARE THE VEGETABLES

Chop the lettuce, halve the tomatoes, slice the olives, and chop the artichoke hearts and roasted red peppers.

STEP 2
PREPARE MEATS AND CHEESE

Chop the salami into bite-sized pieces and cube the provolone cheese.

STEP 3
MAKE THE DRESSING

In a small bowl, whisk together red wine vinegar, olive oil, salt, and pepper.

STEP 4
COMBINE INGREDIENTS

In a large salad bowl, combine the lettuce, tomatoes, olives, artichokes, roasted peppers, salami, provolone, and red onion.

STEP 5
DRESS AND SERVE

Drizzle the dressing over the salad, toss everything to combine, and serve immediately for a burst of Mediterranean flavor.

TY'S ITALIAN ARUGULA SALAD WITH LEMON AND PARMESAN

INGREDIENTS

- 4 cups arugula leaves, washed and dried
- 1/4 cup Parmesan cheese, shaved
- 2 tbsp extra-virgin olive oil
- 1 tbsp freshly squeezed lemon juice
- Salt and pepper to taste
- 1/4 cup toasted pine nuts (optional)

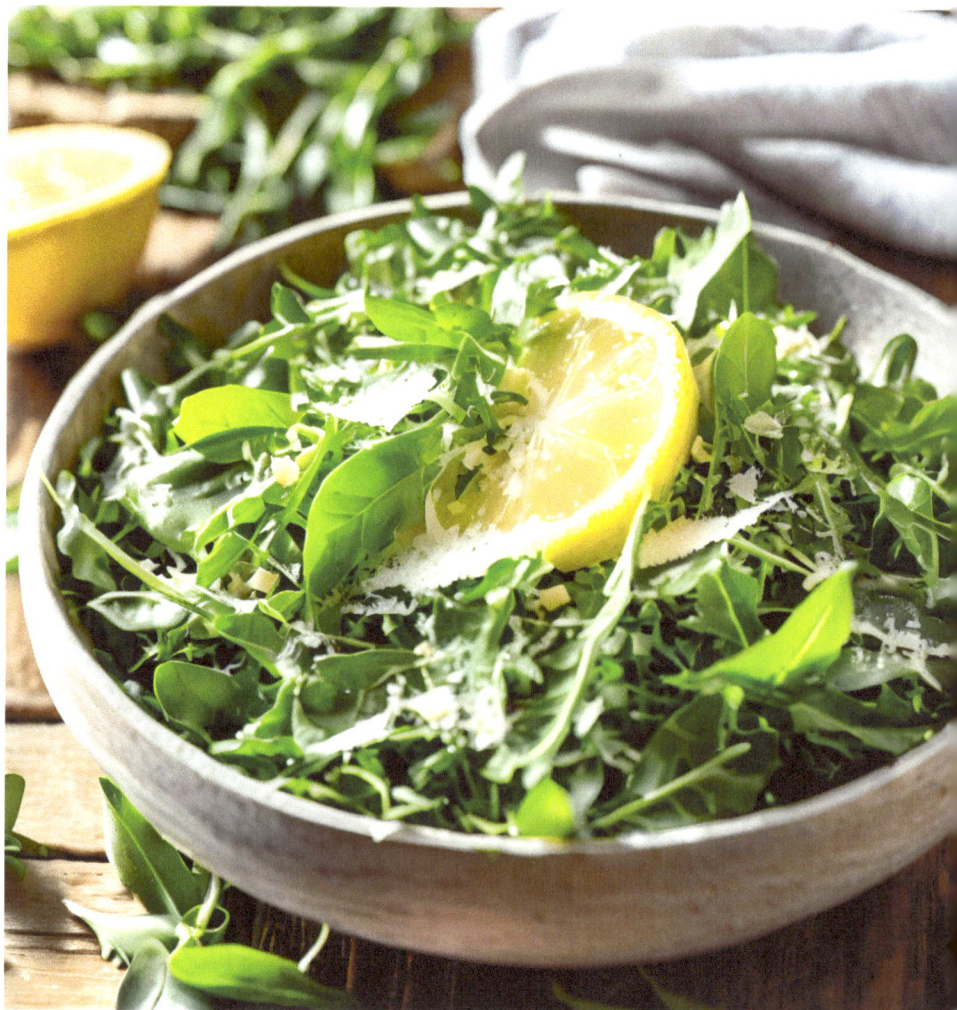

DIRECTIONS

STEP 1
PREPARE THE DRESSING

In a small bowl, whisk together the olive oil, lemon juice, salt, and pepper.

STEP 2
COMBINE INGREDIENTS

Place the arugula in a large bowl. Add the shaved Parmesan and toasted pine nuts, if desired.

STEP 3
DRESS THE SALAD

Drizzle the lemon dressing over the arugula and toss gently to coat.

STEP 4
SERVE IMMEDIATELY

Serve right away to enjoy the peppery arugula with tangy lemon and savory Parmesan.

ITALIAN MARINATED ZUCCHINI SALAD

INGREDIENTS

- 3 medium zucchini, thinly sliced
- 2 tbsp red wine vinegar
- 1/4 cup olive oil
- 2 garlic cloves, minced
- Salt and black pepper to taste
- Fresh basil leaves for garnish

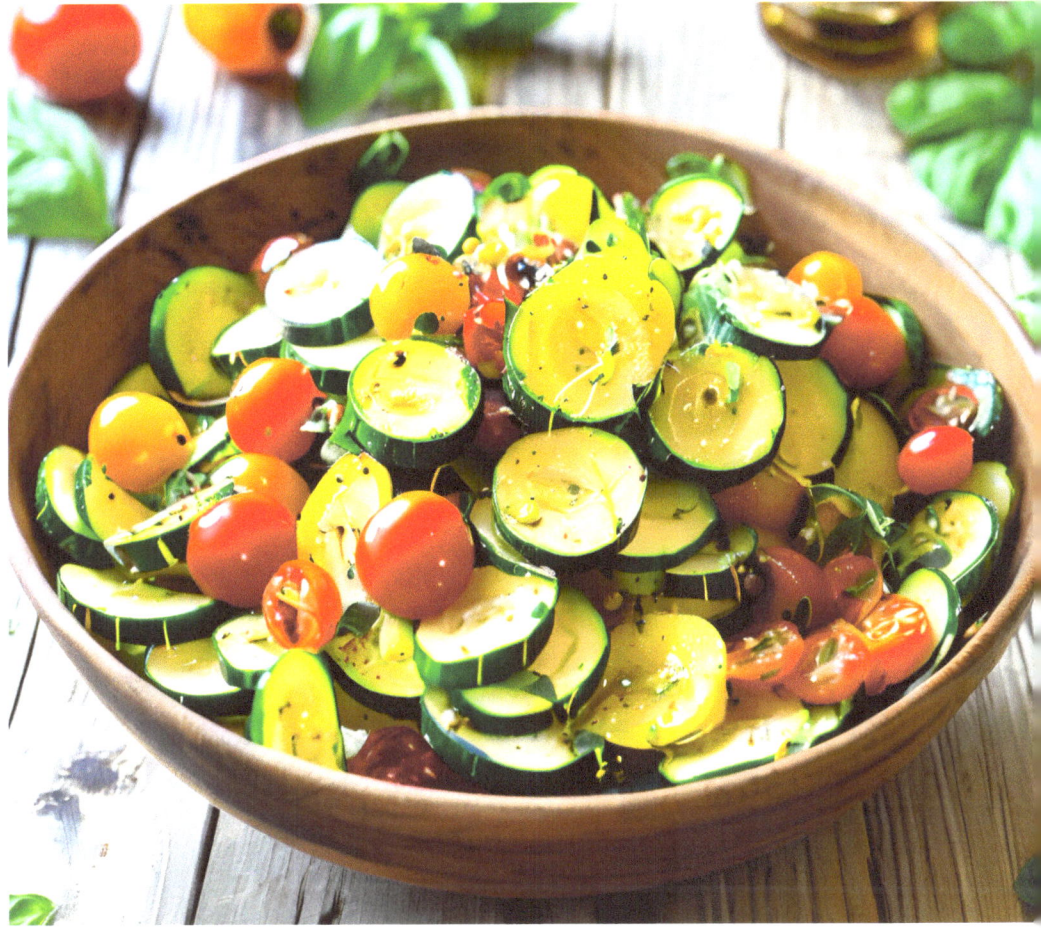

DIRECTIONS

STEP 1
MARINATE THE ZUCCHINI

Place the sliced zucchini in a large bowl. In a separate small bowl, whisk together red wine vinegar, olive oil, minced garlic, salt, and pepper.

STEP 2
COMBINE AND MARINATE

Pour the dressing over the zucchini and toss to coat. Cover the bowl and let it marinate for at least 1 hour in the fridge to allow the flavors to meld.

STEP 3
SERVE

Garnish with fresh basil leaves and serve chilled as a refreshing appetizer.

INSALATA DI FINOCCHI E ARANCE
(FENNEL AND ORANGE SALAD)

INGREDIENTS

- 2 medium fennel bulbs, thinly sliced
- 2 large oranges, peeled and thinly sliced
- 1/4 red onion, thinly sliced
- 1/4 cup black olives, pitted and sliced
- 1/4 cup extra-virgin olive oil
- 2 tbsp white wine vinegar
- Salt and black pepper to taste
- Fresh parsley, chopped, for garnish

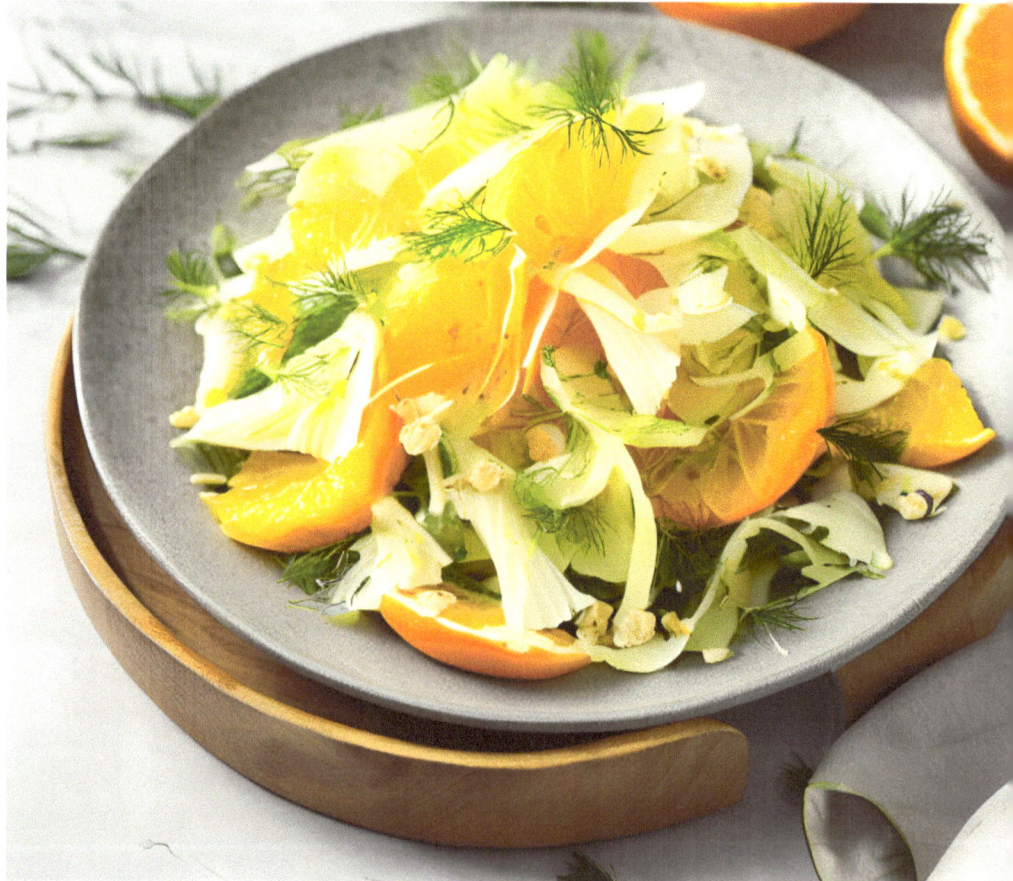

DIRECTIONS

STEP 1
PREPARE THE VEGETABLES

Trim the fennel bulbs, reserving a few of the fronds for garnish. Slice the fennel as thinly as possible (a mandoline works best). Thinly slice the red onion and set aside.

STEP 2
PREPARE THE ORANGES

Slice the top and bottom off each orange, then carefully peel off the skin and pith with a knife. Slice the oranges into thin rounds.

STEP 3
ASSEMBLE THE SALAD

In a large serving bowl or plate, layer the fennel, orange slices, and red onion. Scatter the black olives over the salad.

STEP 4
MAKE THE DRESSING

In a small bowl, whisk together the olive oil, white wine vinegar, salt, and pepper.

STEP 5
DRESS AND GARNISH

Drizzle the dressing over the salad, garnish with chopped parsley and reserved fennel fronds, and serve immediately.

BRESAOLA SALAD WITH ARUGULA AND PARMESAN

INGREDIENTS

- 4 oz bresaola (cured Italian beef), thinly sliced
- 4 cups fresh arugula
- 1/4 cup shaved Parmesan cheese
- 2 tbsp lemon juice
- 3 tbsp extra-virgin olive oil
- Salt and black pepper to taste

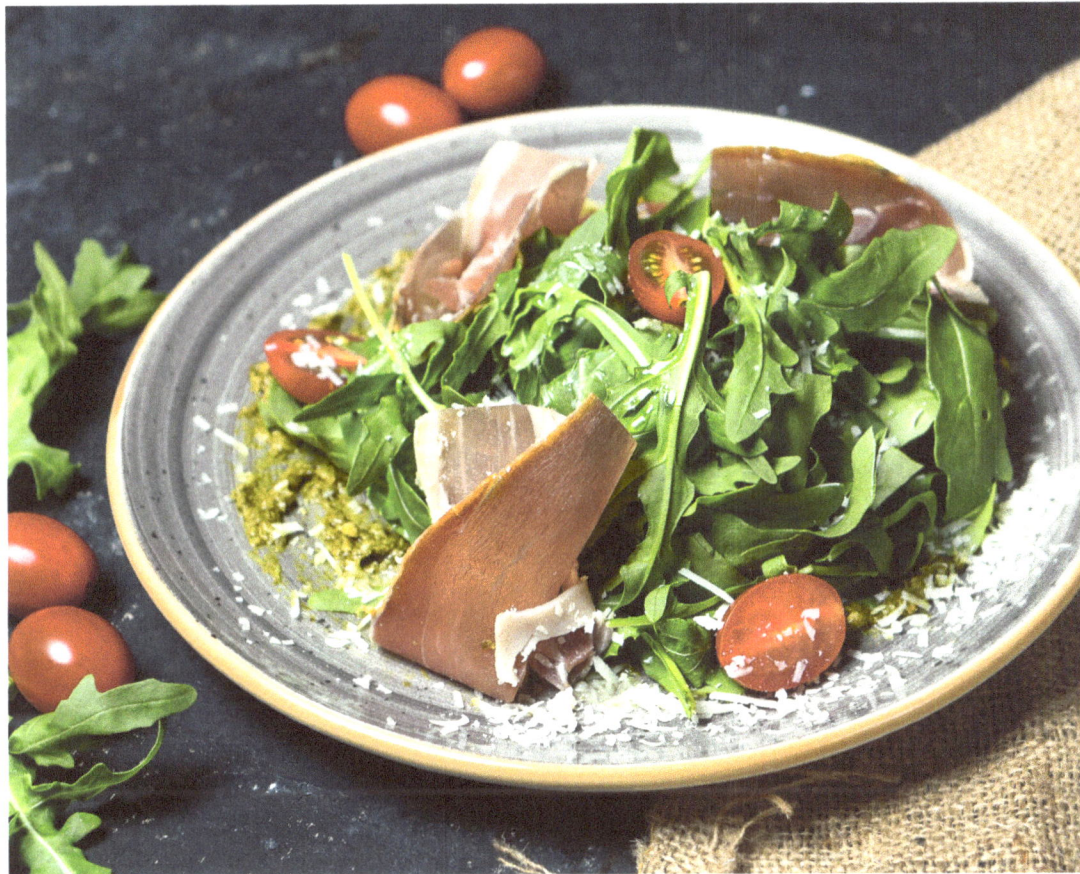

DIRECTIONS

STEP 1
PREPARE THE ARUGULA

Wash and dry the arugula thoroughly, then place it in a large serving bowl or on a platter.

STEP 2
ARRANGE THE BRESAOLA

Lay the thin slices of bresaola over the arugula, distributing them evenly.

STEP 3
ADD THE PARMESAN

Use a vegetable peeler to shave the Parmesan and scatter the shavings over the salad.

STEP 4
MAKE THE DRESSING

In a small bowl, whisk together the lemon juice, olive oil, salt, and pepper.

STEP 5
DRESS AND GARNISH

Drizzle the dressing over the salad and gently toss just before serving. The combination of peppery arugula, salty Parmesan, and tender bresaola makes this a perfect starter or light meal.

ITALIAN CHICKPEA SALAD WITH SUN-DRIED TOMATOES

INGREDIENTS

- 1 can (15 oz) chickpeas, drained and rinsed
- 1/2 cup sun-dried tomatoes, thinly sliced (packed in oil)
- 1/2 cup cherry tomatoes, halved
- 1/2 red onion, finely diced
- 1/4 cup fresh basil leaves, torn
- 1/4 cup fresh parsley, chopped
- 3 tbsp olive oil
- 1 tbsp red wine vinegar
- Salt and black pepper to taste

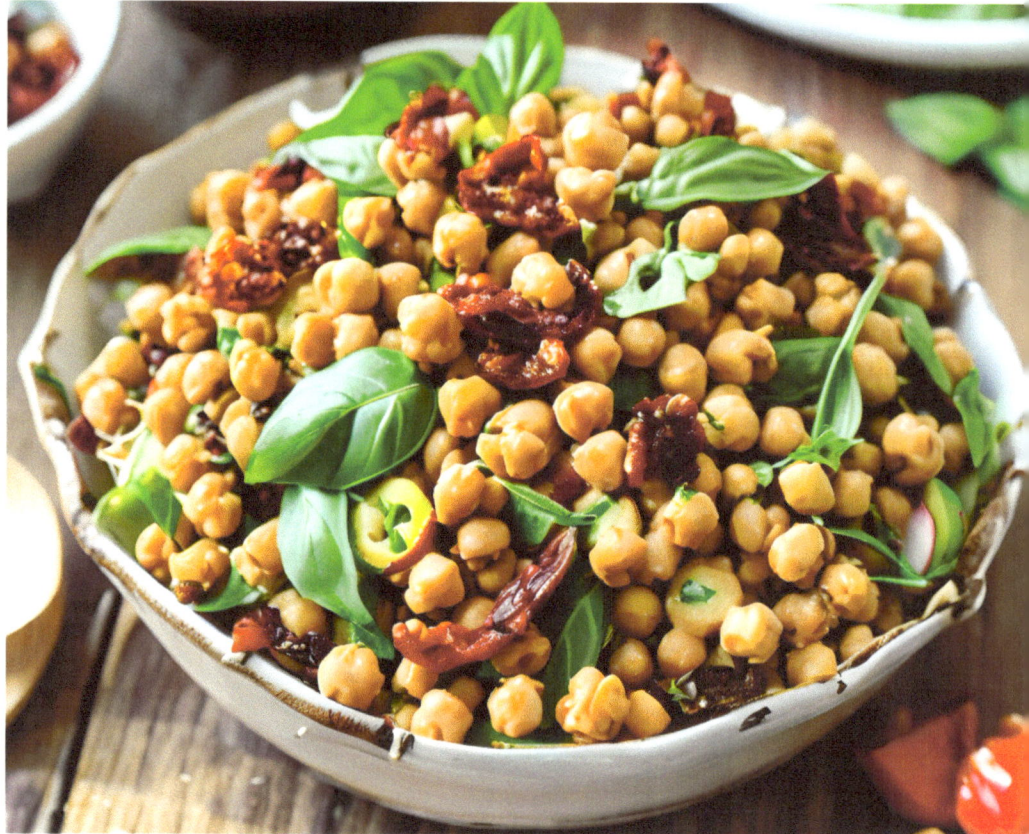

DIRECTIONS

STEP 1
PREPARE THE INGREDIENTS

Rinse and drain the chickpeas, and place them in a large mixing bowl. Thinly slice the sun-dried tomatoes and cherry tomatoes, and finely dice the red onion.

STEP 2
COMBINE THE INGREDIENTS

Add the tomatoes, onion, basil, and parsley to the bowl with the chickpeas.

STEP 3
MAKE THE DRESSING

In a small bowl, whisk together the olive oil, red wine vinegar, salt, and pepper.

STEP 4
TOSS THE SALAD

Pour the dressing over the salad ingredients and toss gently to coat.

STEP 5
SERVE

This salad can be enjoyed immediately or allowed to chill in the refrigerator for a deeper infusion of flavors.

TUSCAN BEAN SALAD WITH FRESH HERBS

INGREDIENTS

- 1 can (15 oz) cannellini beans, drained and rinsed
- 1/2 cup cherry tomatoes, halved
- 1/4 cup red onion, thinly sliced
- 1/4 cup black olives, pitted and sliced
- 1/4 cup fresh parsley, chopped
- 2 tbsp fresh rosemary, chopped
- 1/4 cup extra-virgin olive oil
- 2 tbsp white balsamic vinegar
- Salt and black pepper to taste

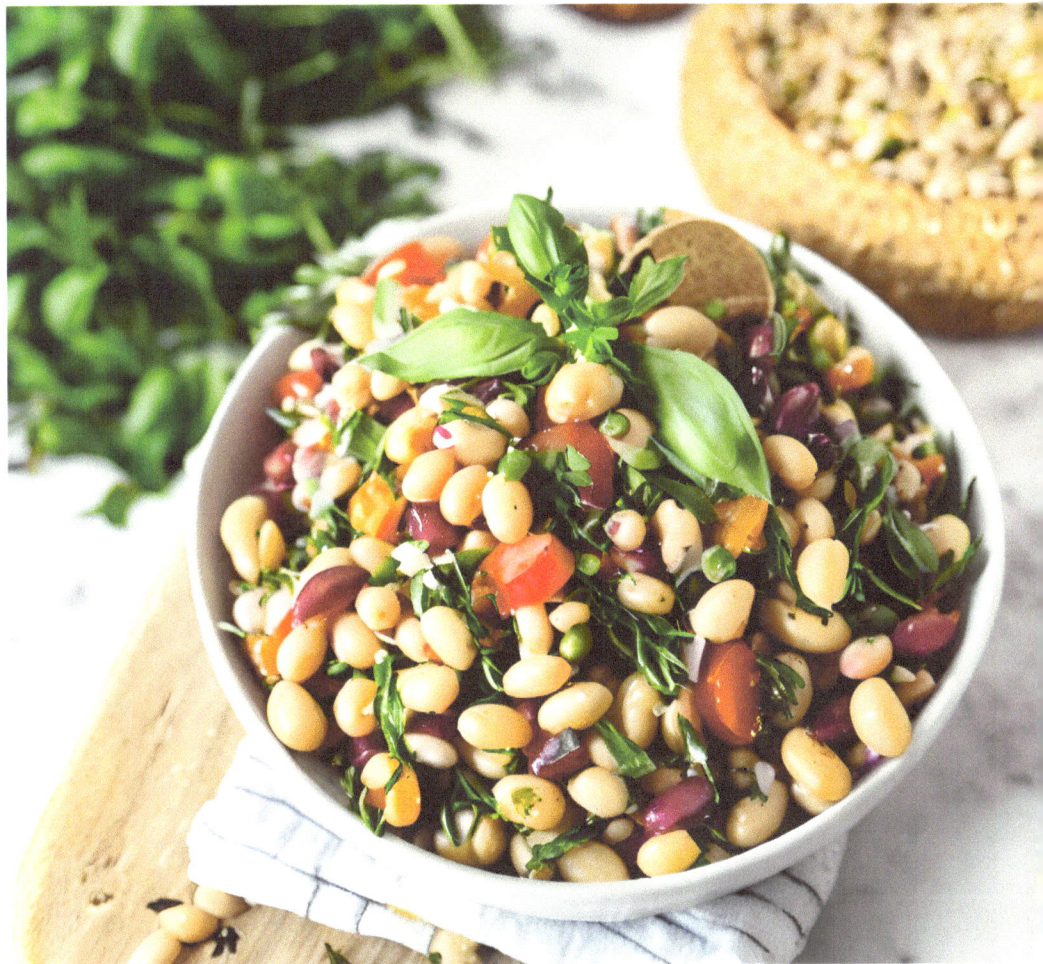

DIRECTIONS

STEP 1
PREPARE THE INGREDIENTS

Rinse and drain the cannellini beans and add them to a large mixing bowl. Halve the cherry tomatoes, thinly slice the red onion, and slice the olives.

STEP 2
ADD FRESH HERBS

Finely chop the parsley and rosemary, and add them to the bowl with the beans and other vegetables.

STEP 3
MAKE THE DRESSING

In a small bowl, whisk together the olive oil, white balsamic vinegar, salt, and pepper.

STEP 4
COMBINE AND TOSS

Pour the dressing over the salad and toss everything together gently.

STEP 5
SERVE

Let the salad sit for a few minutes to allow the flavors to meld, or refrigerate for up to an hour for a more pronounced taste. This refreshing salad pairs wonderfully with grilled meats or as a standalone dish.

PASTA

PASTA CARBONARA

INGREDIENTS

- 12 oz spaghetti
- 4 oz pancetta or guanciale, diced
- 2 large eggs
- 1 cup Pecorino Romano cheese, finely grated
- Salt and black pepper, to taste

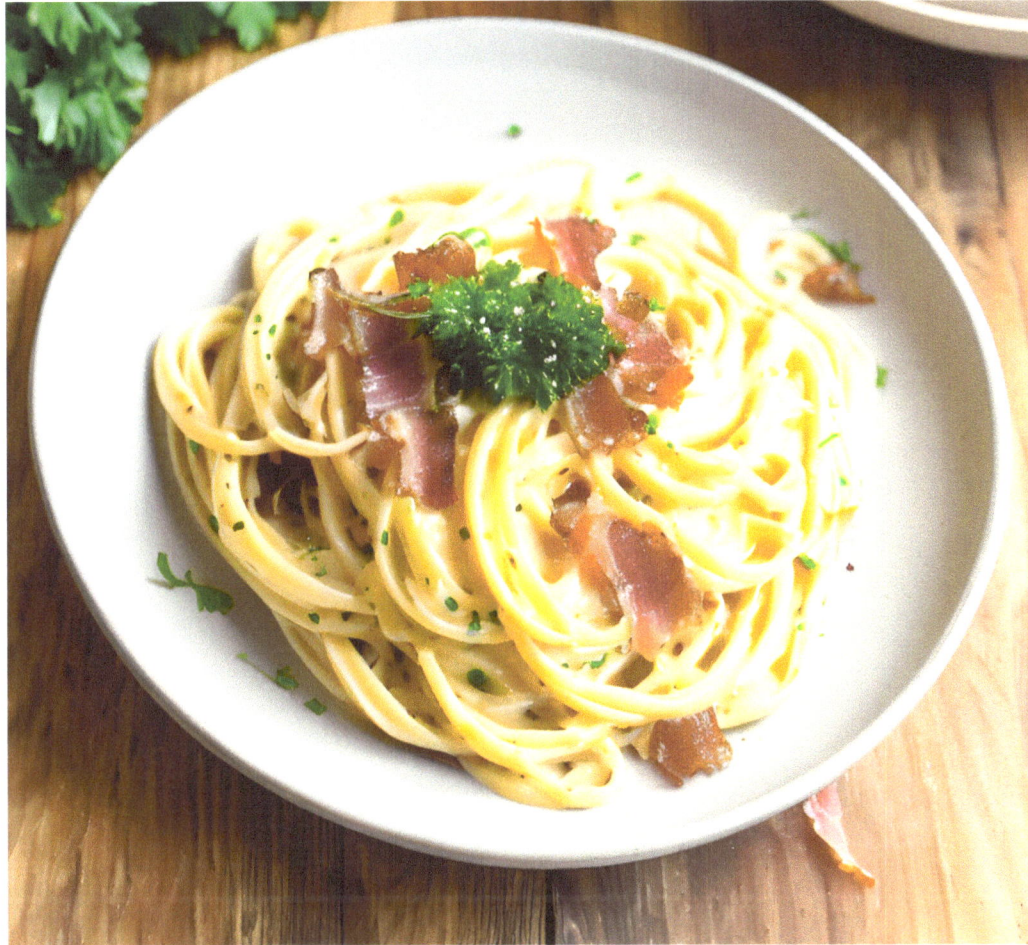

DIRECTIONS

STEP 1
COOK THE PASTA

Bring a large pot of salted water to a boil and cook the spaghetti according to the package instructions, usually for about 9-10 minutes, until al dente. Reserve about 1/2 cup of pasta cooking water before draining.

STEP 2
PREPARE THE PANCETTA

Heat a large skillet over medium heat. Add the diced pancetta (or guanciale) and cook, stirring occasionally, until crispy, about 5-7 minutes. Remove from heat once crispy.

STEP 3
PREPARE THE SAUCE

In a separate bowl, whisk the eggs and Pecorino Romano cheese together until well combined. Add freshly ground black pepper to taste. This will form the creamy base of your carbonara.

STEP 4
COMBINE PASTA AND PANCETTA

Once the pasta is drained, immediately toss it into the pan with the pancetta, letting the residual heat from the pasta slightly cool the pancetta and begin to melt the fat. Stir the pasta and pancetta well to coat the noodles.

STEP 5
ADD THE EGG MIXTURE

Slowly pour the egg and cheese mixture over the pasta while continuously tossing the pasta to prevent the eggs from scrambling. Add reserved pasta water a little at a time if the mixture feels too thick.

STEP 6
SERVE

Once the sauce has formed a creamy texture that coats the pasta, season with more pepper and serve immediately, topped with extra Pecorino Romano.

RIGATONI BOLOGNESE
(TOPPED WITH A DOLLOP OF RICOTTA CHEESE)

- 12 oz rigatoni or penne
- 1 large eggplant, cubed
- 3 tbsp olive oil
- 2 garlic cloves, minced
- 1 can (14 oz) crushed tomatoes
- Fresh basil leaves
- Salt, pepper, and crushed red pepper flakes, to taste
- Ricotta Salata cheese, for garnish

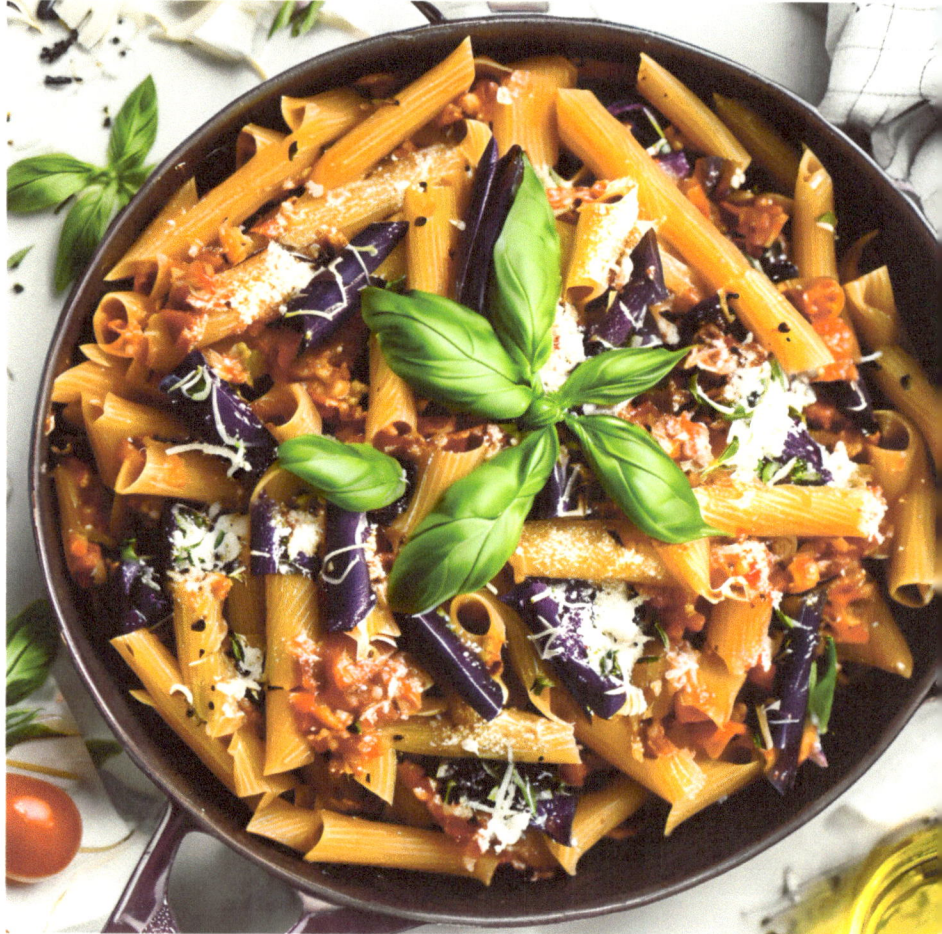

DIRECTIONS

STEP 1
PREPARE THE EGGPLANT
Cube the eggplant into bite-sized pieces. Place them in a colander, sprinkle with salt, and let them sit for 20-30 minutes to draw out excess moisture. Pat dry with a paper towel.

STEP 2
COOK THE EGGPLANT
Heat olive oil in a large pan over medium-high heat. Once hot, add the eggplant cubes in batches and sauté until they are golden brown on all sides, about 10-12 minutes. Remove from the pan and set aside.

STEP 3
PREPARE THE SAUCE
In the same pan, lower the heat and add the minced garlic. Cook for about 1 minute until fragrant, then add the crushed tomatoes. Simmer the sauce for 15-20 minutes, allowing it to reduce slightly. Season with salt, pepper, and crushed red pepper flakes for a slight kick.

STEP 4
COOK THE PASTA
In a large pot of salted boiling water, cook the pasta until al dente, according to package instructions. Drain the pasta, reserving about 1/2 cup of pasta water.

STEP 5
COMBINE
Add the cooked pasta to the pan with the tomato sauce, stirring to coat. Add the eggplant back into the pan and toss everything together. If the sauce is too thick, add a splash of reserved pasta water to achieve the desired consistency.

STEP 6
SERVE
Garnish with fresh basil leaves and crumble Ricotta Salata cheese over the top before serving.

SPAGHETTI AGLIO E OLIO

INGREDIENTS

- 12 oz spaghetti
- 1/4 cup olive oil
- 4 garlic cloves, thinly sliced
- 1/2 tsp red pepper flakes
- Salt and black pepper, to taste
- Fresh parsley, chopped

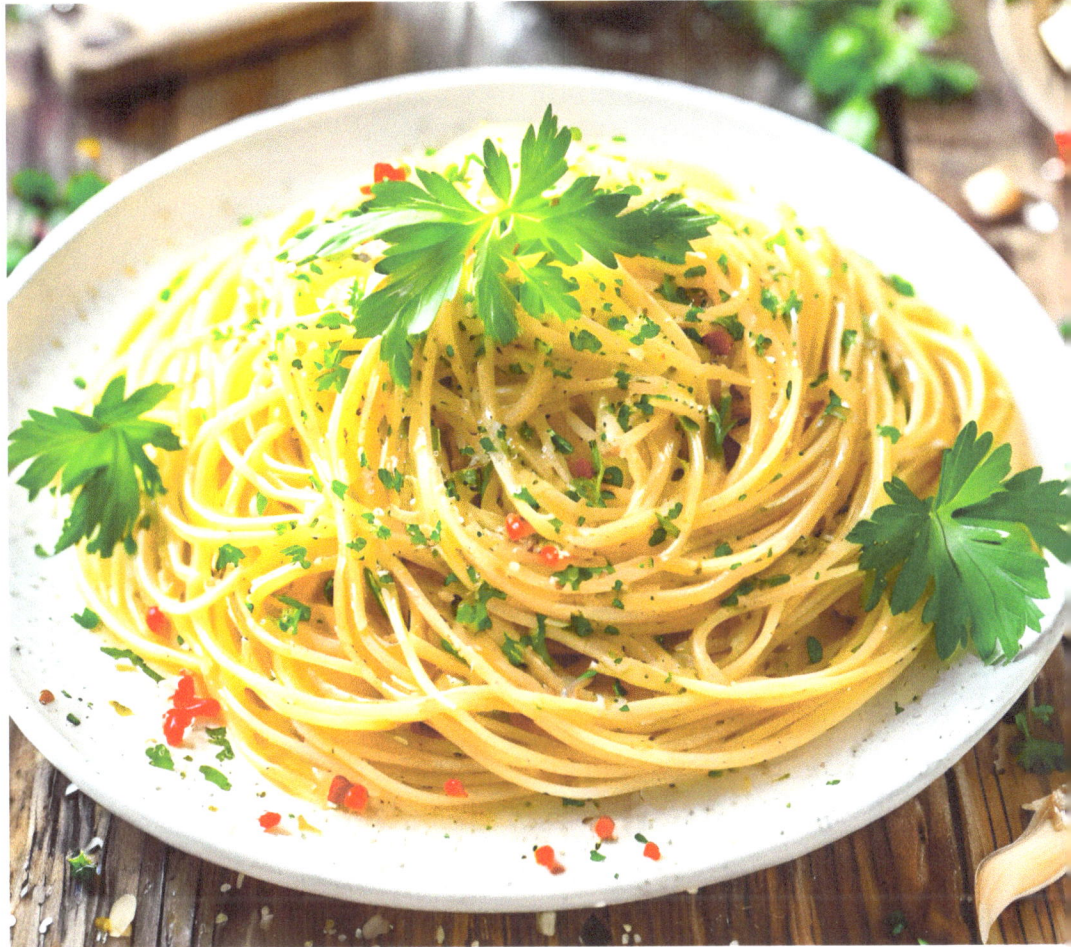

DIRECTIONS

STEP 1
COOK THE PASTA

Bring a large pot of salted water to a boil. Cook the spaghetti for 9-10 minutes until al dente, then drain, reserving about 1/2 cup of pasta water.

STEP 2
PREPARE THE AGLIO E OLIO SAUCE

In a large pan, heat the olive oil over medium heat. Add the garlic slices and sauté, stirring constantly, for about 2 minutes until the garlic becomes golden and fragrant, but not browned (as it will become bitter).

STEP 3
ADD THE RED PEPPER FLAKES

Stir in the red pepper flakes and cook for another 30 seconds to release their flavor.

STEP 4
COMBINE PASTA AND SAUCE

Add the cooked spaghetti to the pan with the garlic oil. Toss everything together, adding reserved pasta water little by little to help coat the spaghetti in the oil and garlic mixture.

STEP 5
SERVE

Season with salt and pepper to taste. Garnish with freshly chopped parsley and serve immediately.

PASTA PRIMAVERA

INGREDIENTS

- 12 oz fettuccine
- 1/4 cup olive oil
- 1/2 cup cherry tomatoes, halved
- 1 zucchini, sliced
- 1 yellow bell pepper, sliced
- 1/2 cup peas
- Fresh basil
- Salt and pepper, to taste
- Parmesan cheese, grated

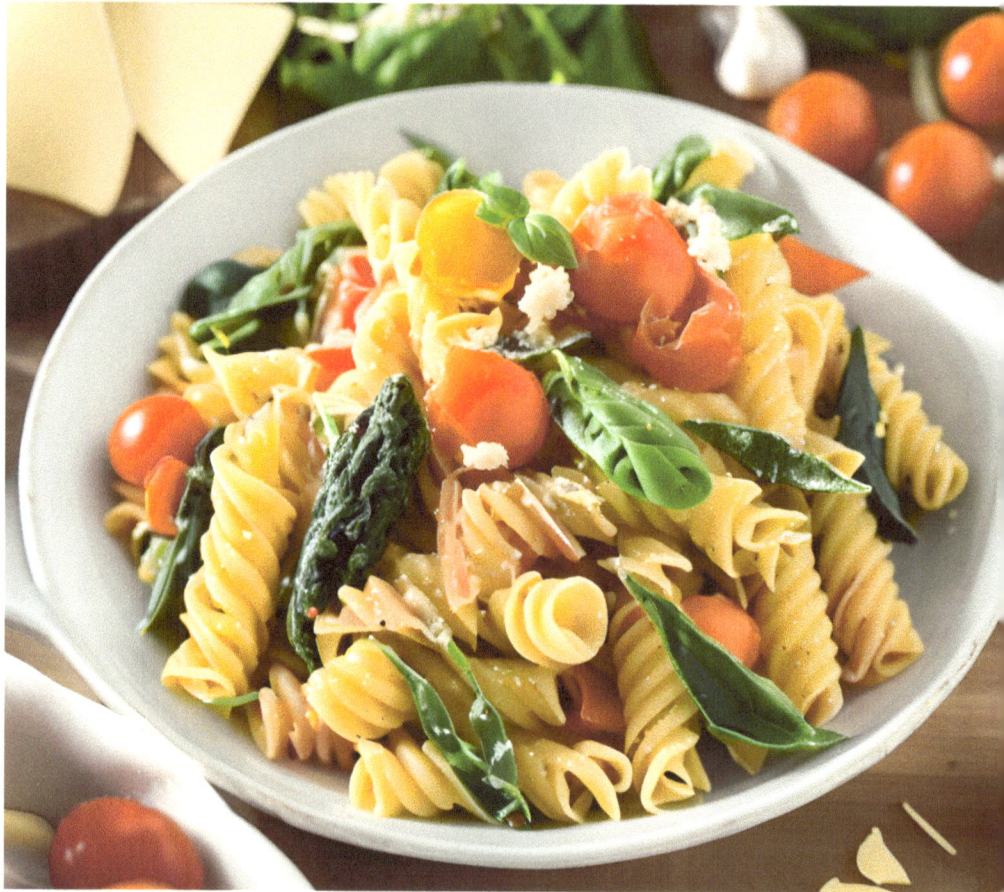

DIRECTIONS

STEP 1
COOK THE PASTA

Bring a large pot of salted water to a boil. Cook the fettuccine until al dente, usually about 8-9 minutes, then drain and set aside.

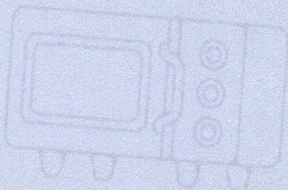

STEP 2
PREPARE THE VEGETABLES

Heat olive oil in a large pan over medium-high heat. Add the zucchini, bell pepper, and peas, sautéing for about 5-7 minutes until just tender. Add the halved cherry tomatoes and cook for an additional 2-3 minutes until they soften.

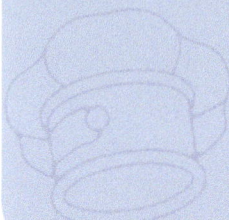

STEP 3
COMBINE THE PASTA AND VEGETABLES

Add the cooked fettuccine to the pan with the vegetables and toss everything together until well combined.

STEP 4
SEASON AND SERVE

Season with salt, pepper, and fresh basil to taste. Garnish with a generous amount of grated Parmesan cheese before serving.

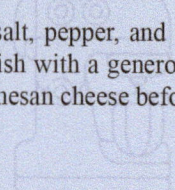

RED CLAM SAUCE

- 12 oz linguine
- 2 tbsp olive oil
- 3 garlic cloves, minced
- 1/2 cup white wine
- 1 lb clams, scrubbed and rinsed
- Fresh parsley, chopped
- Salt and pepper, to taste
- 16oz. crushed tomato

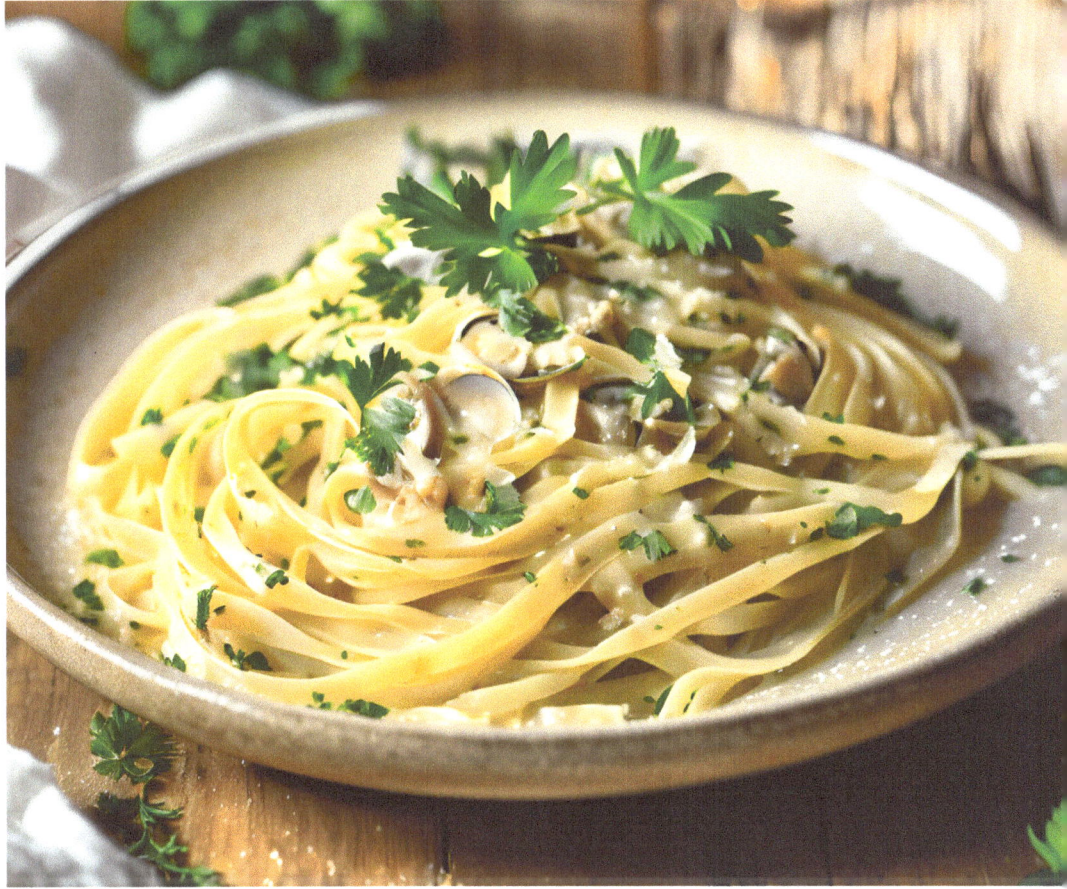

DIRECTIONS

STEP 1
COOK THE PASTA

In a large pot of salted water, cook the linguine until al dente, about 9-10 minutes. Drain, reserving some pasta water for later.

STEP 2
PREPARE THE CLAM SAUCE

Heat olive oil in a large pan over medium heat. Add minced garlic and sauté until fragrant, about 1 minute. Pour in the white wine, and allow it to simmer for 2-3 minutes to reduce slightly tomatoes.

STEP 3
COOK THE CLAMS

Add the clams to the pan and cover. Cook for 5-7 minutes or until all the clams have opened. Discard any that remain closed.

STEP 4
COMBINE PASTA AND SAUCE

Add the drained linguine to the pan with the clams. Toss to combine, adding a bit of reserved pasta water to help coat the pasta in the sauce.

STEP 5
SERVE

Season with salt and pepper to taste. Garnish with freshly chopped parsley and serve immediately.

These detailed steps should guide you through creating some classic Italian pasta dishes with precision and flavor. Enjoy your cooking!

MOM'S LASAGNA ALLA BOLOGNESE
(RED SAUCE)

- 1 lb ground beef
- 1/2 lb ground Italian pork sausage
- 1 medium onion, chopped
- 2 garlic cloves, minced
- 1 carrot, grated
- 1 celery stalk, chopped
- 1 can (22 oz) crushed tomatoes
- 1 cup red wine
- 9-12 lasagna noodles
- 2 cups cups marinara sauce (tomato,garlic,basil)
- 1 1/2 cups grated mozzarella
- 1/2 cup Parmesan cheese
- 1 1/2 cups ricotta

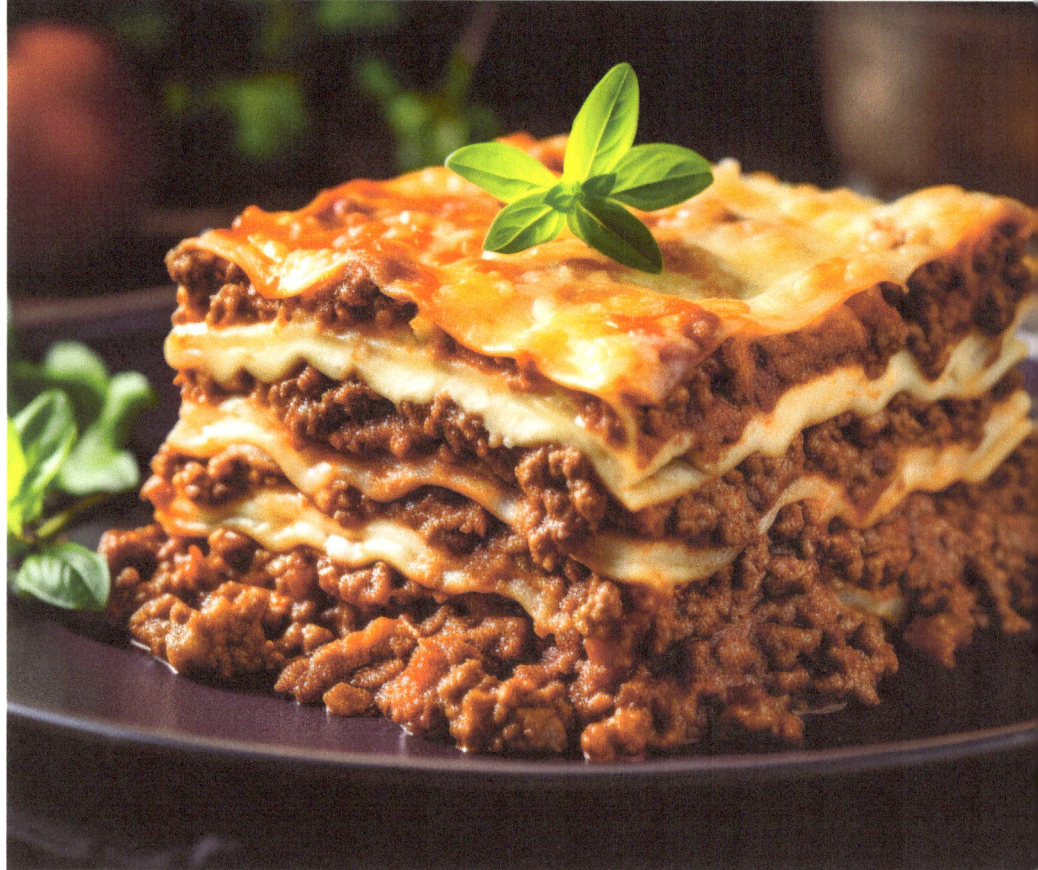

DIRECTIONS

STEP 1
PREPARE THE BOLOGNESE SAUCE

In a large pot, heat olive oil over medium heat. Add the onion, carrot, and celery, cooking for about 5 minutes until softened. Add the minced garlic, ground beef, and sausage, breaking up the meat with a spoon, and cook until browned.

STEP 2
DEGLAZE

Pour in the red wine and let it reduce by half, about 4 minutes. Add the crushed tomatoes, salt, and pepper. Simmer for at least 1 hour, stirring occasionally.

STEP 3
PREPARE THE LASAGNA NOODLES

Cook the lasagna noodles according to the package instructions. Drain and set aside.

STEP 4
ASSEMBLE THE LASAGNA

Preheat your oven to 375°F (190°C). In a baking dish, layer the Bolognese sauce, followed by a layer of lasagna noodles, then some ricotta, parmesan, mozzarella mix. Repeat the layers and finish with marinara sauce and shredded mozzarella.

STEP 5
BAKE AND SERVE

Cover with foil and bake for 30 minutes. Remove the foil and bake for an additional 15 minutes until bubbly and golden. Let it rest for 10 minutes before slicing.

PENNE ARRABBIATA

INGREDIENTS

- 12 oz penne pasta
- 1/4 cup olive oil
- 4 garlic cloves, sliced thin
- 1-2 tsp red pepper flakes (to taste)
- 1 can (14 oz) crushed tomatoes
- Salt and pepper, to taste
- Fresh parsley, chopped

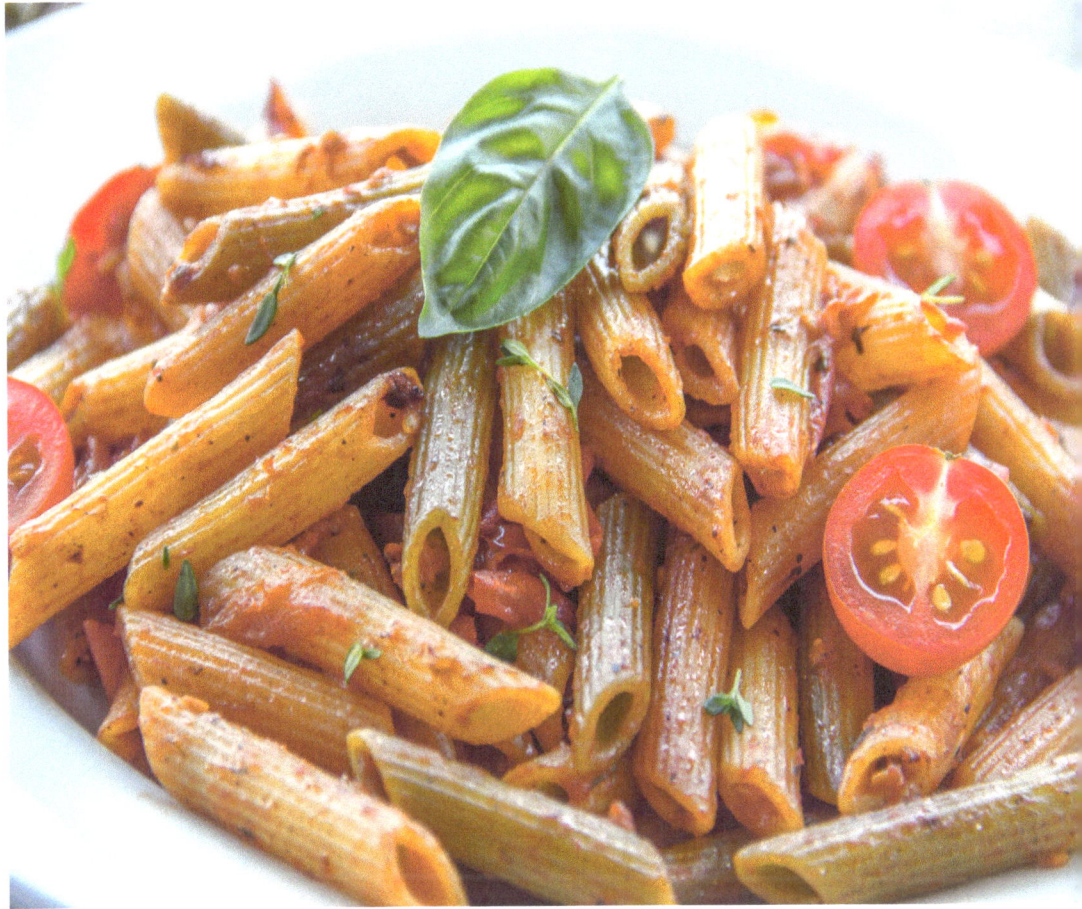

DIRECTIONS

STEP 1
COOK THE PASTA

Bring a large pot of salted water to a boil and cook the penne according to package instructions, about 9-10 minutes, until al dente.

STEP 2
MAKE THE SAUCE

While the pasta cooks, heat olive oil in a large pan over medium heat. Add the sliced garlic and sauté until golden, about 1-2 minutes, being careful not to burn the garlic.

STEP 3
ADD THE RED PEPPER FLAKES

Add the red pepper flakes to the pan and cook for 30 seconds.

STEP 4
SIMMER THE TOMATOES

Pour in the crushed tomatoes and season with salt and pepper. Simmer the sauce for 10-15 minutes, allowing the flavors to meld.

STEP 5
COMBINE

Add the cooked pasta directly into the sauce, tossing well to coat. If needed, add a bit of reserved pasta water to help mix everything together.

STEP 6
SERVE

Garnish with fresh chopped parsley and serve hot.

FETTUCCINE ALFREDO

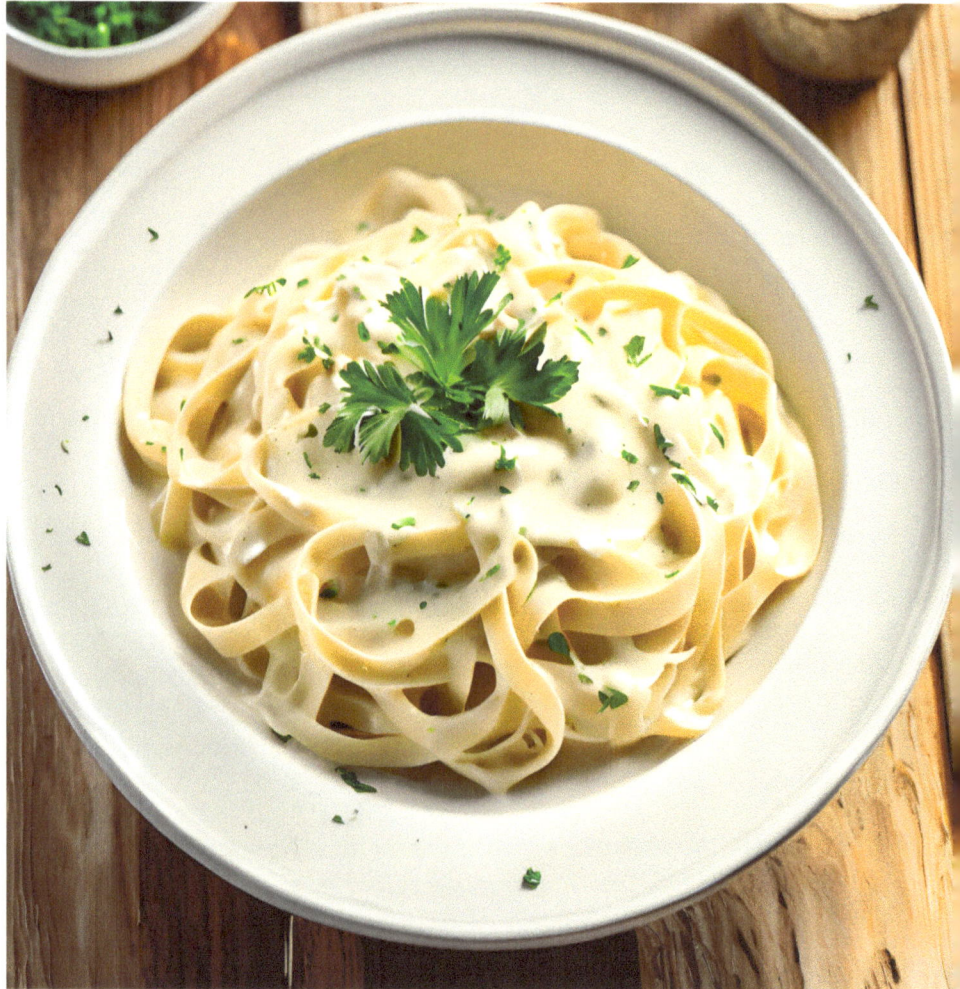

INGREDIENTS

- 12 oz fettuccine
- 1/2 cup unsalted butter
- 1 cup heavy cream
- 2 cups grated Parmesan cheese
- Salt and pepper, to taste
- Fresh parsley, chopped (optional)

DIRECTIONS

STEP 1
COOK THE PASTA

Bring a large pot of salted water to a boil. Add the fettuccine and cook until al dente, about 8-9 minutes. Drain, reserving about 1/2 cup of pasta water.

STEP 2
PREPARE THE ALFREDO SAUCE

In a large skillet, melt the butter over medium heat. Add the heavy cream and bring to a simmer. Stir continuously and let it cook for 3-4 minutes until slightly thickened.

STEP 3
ADD THE CHEESE

Stir in the grated Parmesan cheese, a little at a time, until the sauce becomes creamy and smooth. Season with salt and pepper to taste.

STEP 4
COMBINE THE PASTA AND SAUCE

Add the cooked fettuccine to the sauce, tossing to coat. Add reserved pasta water as needed to adjust the sauce's consistency.

STEP 5
SERVE

Garnish with fresh parsley and extra Parmesan cheese. Serve immediately.

PASTA PUTTANESCA

INGREDIENTS

- 12 oz spaghetti
- 1/4 cup olive oil
- 4 garlic cloves, minced
- 1/4 tsp red pepper flakes
- 1 can (14 oz) diced tomatoes
- 1/4 cup black olives, pitted and chopped
- 2 tbsp capers
- 2 anchovy fillets (optional)
- Fresh parsley, chopped

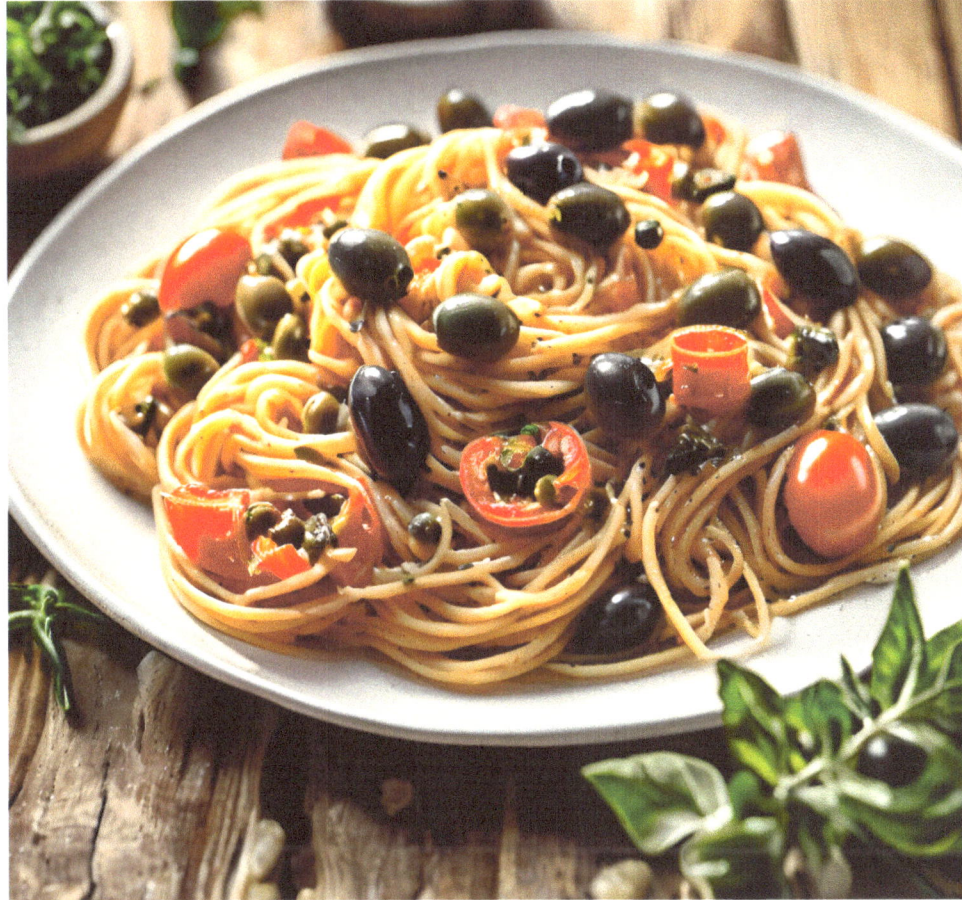

DIRECTIONS

STEP 1
COOK THE PASTA

Bring a pot of salted water to a boil. Cook the spaghetti according to the package instructions, about 9-10 minutes, until al dente. Drain, reserving some pasta water.

STEP 2
MAKE THE SAUCE

In a large pan, heat olive oil over medium heat. Add the minced garlic and red pepper flakes, cooking for 1-2 minutes until the garlic becomes fragrant.

STEP 3
ADD TOMATOES AND SEASONINGS

Stir in the diced tomatoes, olives, capers, and anchovy fillets. Simmer for about 10 minutes, allowing the flavors to meld and the sauce to thicken slightly.

STEP 4
COMBINE THE PASTA

Add the drained spaghetti to the sauce and toss everything together, adding pasta water as needed to help coat the pasta.

STEP 5
SERVE

Garnish with freshly chopped parsley and serve hot.

TORTELLINI IN BRODO

- 1 lb fresh tortellini (cheese or meat)
- 4 cups chicken or vegetable broth
- 1 carrot, peeled and diced
- 1 celery stalk, diced
- 1 small onion, diced
- Salt and pepper, to taste
- Fresh Parmesan, grated (optional)

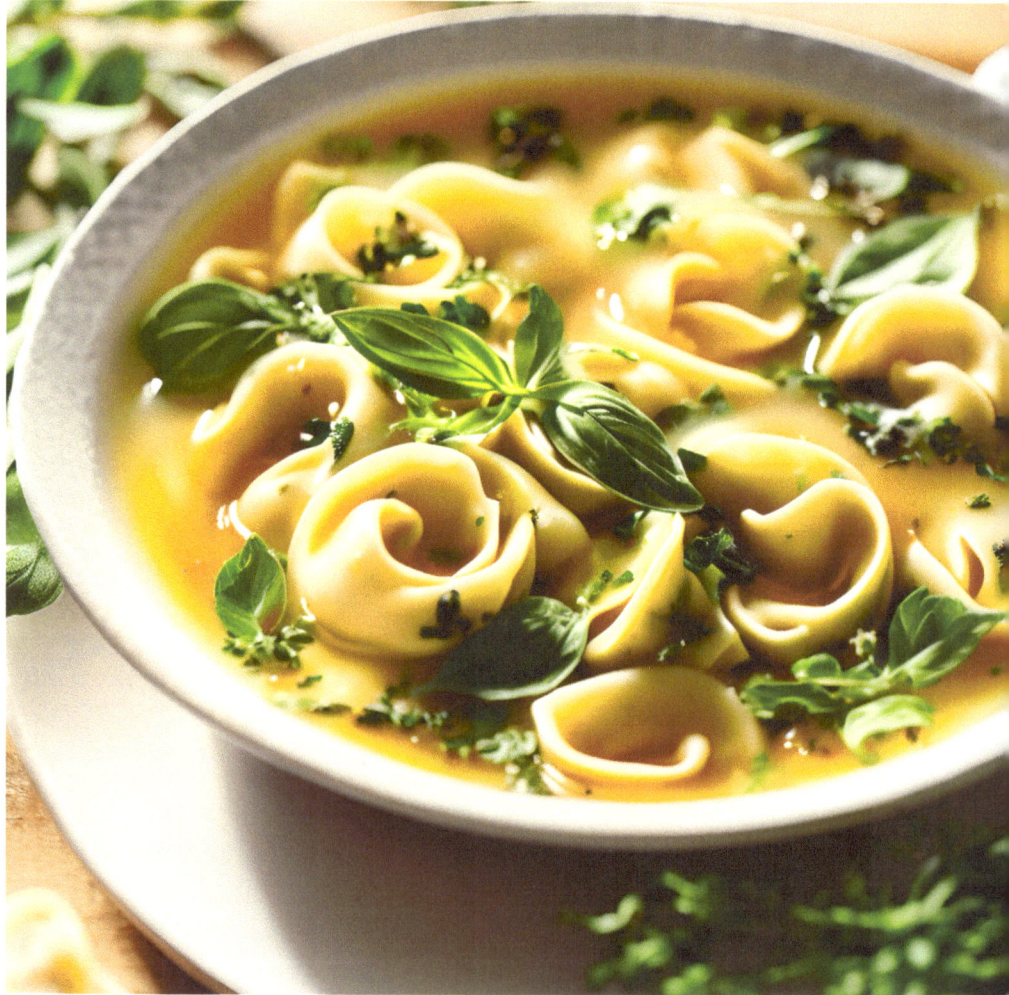

DIRECTIONS

STEP 1
PREPARE THE BROTH

In a large pot, bring the chicken or vegetable broth to a simmer. Add the diced carrot, celery, and onion. Season with salt and pepper and let the broth cook for 15-20 minutes to allow the vegetables to soften and the flavors to develop.

STEP 4
COMBINE THE PASTA

Add the drained spaghetti to the sauce and toss everything together, adding pasta water as needed to help coat the pasta.

STEP 2
COOK THE TORTELLINI

Add the fresh tortellini to the broth and cook according to the package instructions, usually about 3-5 minutes for fresh tortellini.

STEP 5
SERVE

Garnish with freshly chopped parsley and serve hot.

STEP 3
SERVE

Once the tortellini are cooked and floating in the broth, ladle the soup into bowls. Garnish with grated Parmesan cheese if desired and serve immediately.

ENTREES

OSSO BUCO ALLA MILANESE

A traditional Milanese dish made with braised veal shanks cooked in a rich, aromatic sauce of white wine, stock, garlic, onions, carrots, celery, and tomatoes. It's typically served with risotto alla Milanese.

INGREDIENTS

- 4 veal shanks
- 1/2 cup flour (for dredging)
- 1 cup white wine
- 2 cups beef or chicken stock
- 2 tbsp tomato paste
- 1 onion, finely chopped
- 1 carrot, chopped
- 1 celery stalk, chopped
- 2 garlic cloves, minced
- 2 tbsp fresh parsley, chopped
- 1 lemon (for gremolata)
- Salt and pepper, to taste

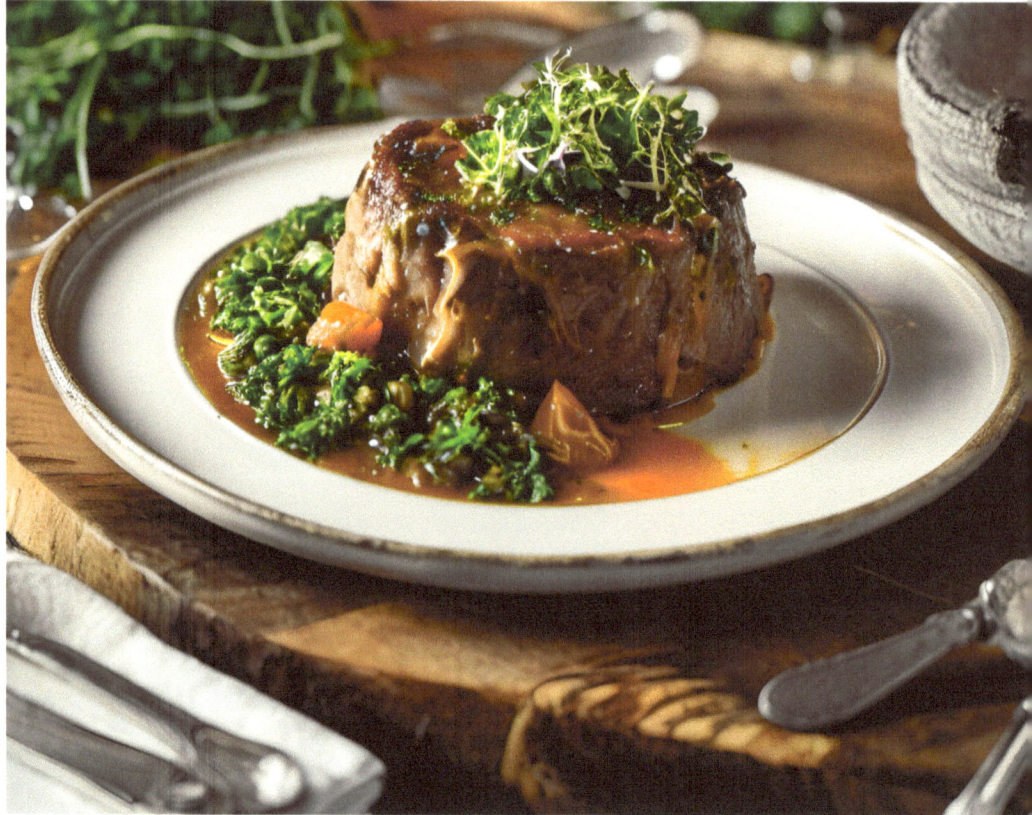

DIRECTIONS

STEP 1
Brown the veal shanks in flour, salt, and pepper.

STEP 2
In a large pot, sauté onions, carrots, celery, and garlic until soft. Add tomato paste and cook briefly.

STEP 3
Add white wine and stock to deglaze, simmering for 30 minutes.

STEP 4
Return veal shanks to the pot, cover, and cook on low for about 2 hours.

STEP 5
Prepare gremolata by combining lemon zest, garlic, and parsley.

STEP 6
Serve hot with gremolata sprinkled on top

CHICKEN PICCATA

A simple, yet elegant dish where chicken breasts are pan-fried, then served in a lemony caper sauce.

INGREDIENTS

- 4 boneless, skinless chicken breasts
- 1/2 cup flour
- 3 tbsp butter
- 1/4 cup white wine
- 2 tbsp lemon juice
- 1/4 cup capers, drained
- Fresh parsley, chopped

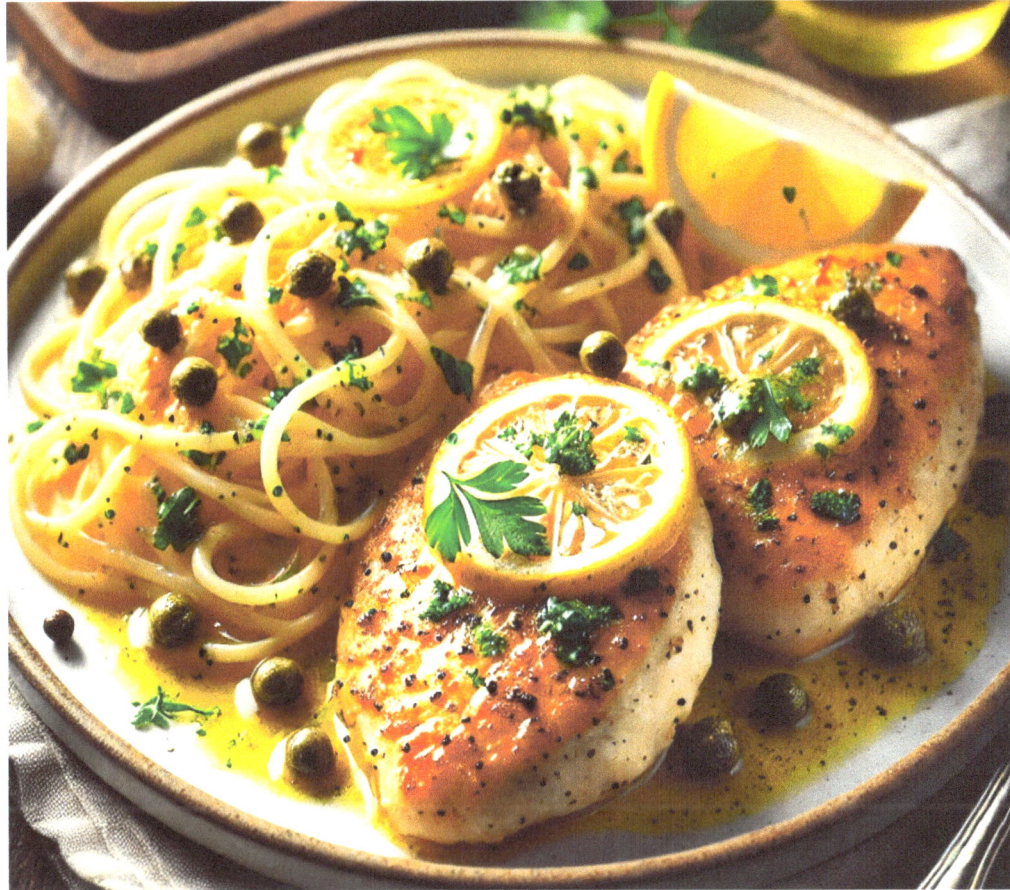

DIRECTIONS

STEP 1

Season chicken breasts, dredge in flour, and fry in butter until golden.

STEP 2

Remove chicken, add wine, lemon juice, and capers to the pan, reducing to a sauce.

STEP 3

Return chicken to the pan, simmering for 10 minutes to absorb the flavors.

STEP 4

Serve with fresh parsley.

EGGPLANT PARMESAN
(MELANZANE ALLA PARMIGIANA)

A classic Italian dish consisting of layers of breaded, fried eggplant slices, marinara sauce, mozzarella, and Parmesan, baked until bubbly and golden.

INGREDIENTS

- 2 large eggplants, peeled, sliced
- 2 cups marinara sauce
- 1 1/2 cups mozzarella cheese
- 1/2 cup grated Parmesan cheese
- 2 eggs, beaten
- 2 cups breadcrumbs
- Olive oil for frying

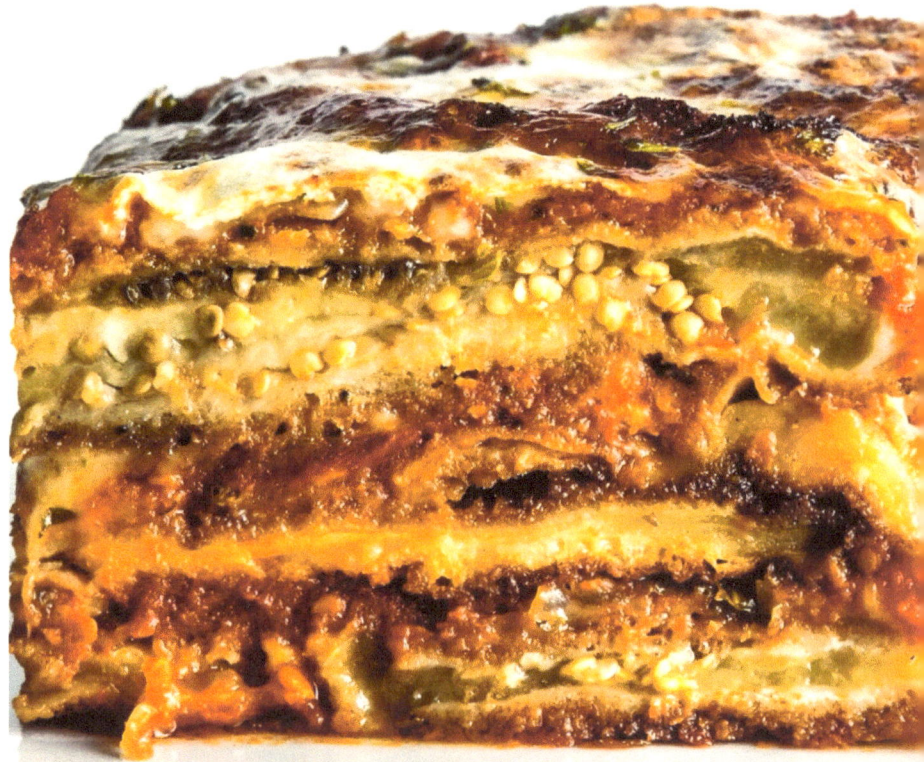

DIRECTIONS

STEP 1

Slice eggplants, salt them, and let them sit to release moisture.

STEP 2

Dip eggplant slices in beaten egg, then breadcrumbs, frying until golden.

STEP 3

In a baking dish, layer fried eggplant, marinara, mozzarella, and Parmesan.

STEP 4

Bake at 375°F for 30 minutes.

BISTECCA ALLA FIORENTINA

A Florentine steak, typically served as a large T-bone, cooked simply over high heat and seasoned with salt, pepper, and olive oil.

INGREDIENTS

- 1 large T-bone steak (about 2 inches thick)
- Olive oil
- Sea salt and black pepper
- Fresh rosemary

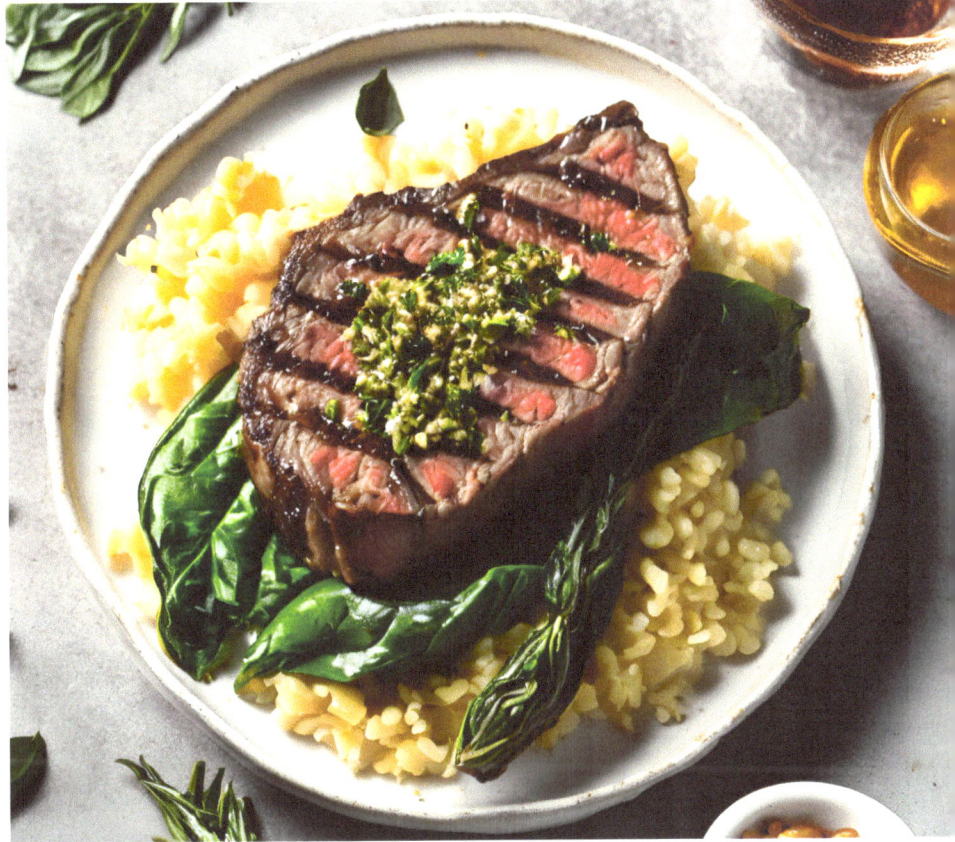

DIRECTIONS

STEP 1
Season steak generously with salt, pepper, and rosemary.

STEP 2
Grill over high heat for about 5 minutes per side, depending on desired doneness.

STEP 3
Rest the steak for 5 minutes before slicing.

RISOTTO ALLA MILANESE

A luxurious rice dish cooked in a saffron-infused broth, creating a creamy texture and golden color.

INGREDIENTS

- 1 1/2 cups Arborio rice
- 1/2 onion, chopped
- 1/4 cup dry white wine
- 4 cups chicken stock
- 1/2 tsp saffron threads
- 1/4 cup Parmesan cheese
- 3 tbsp butter

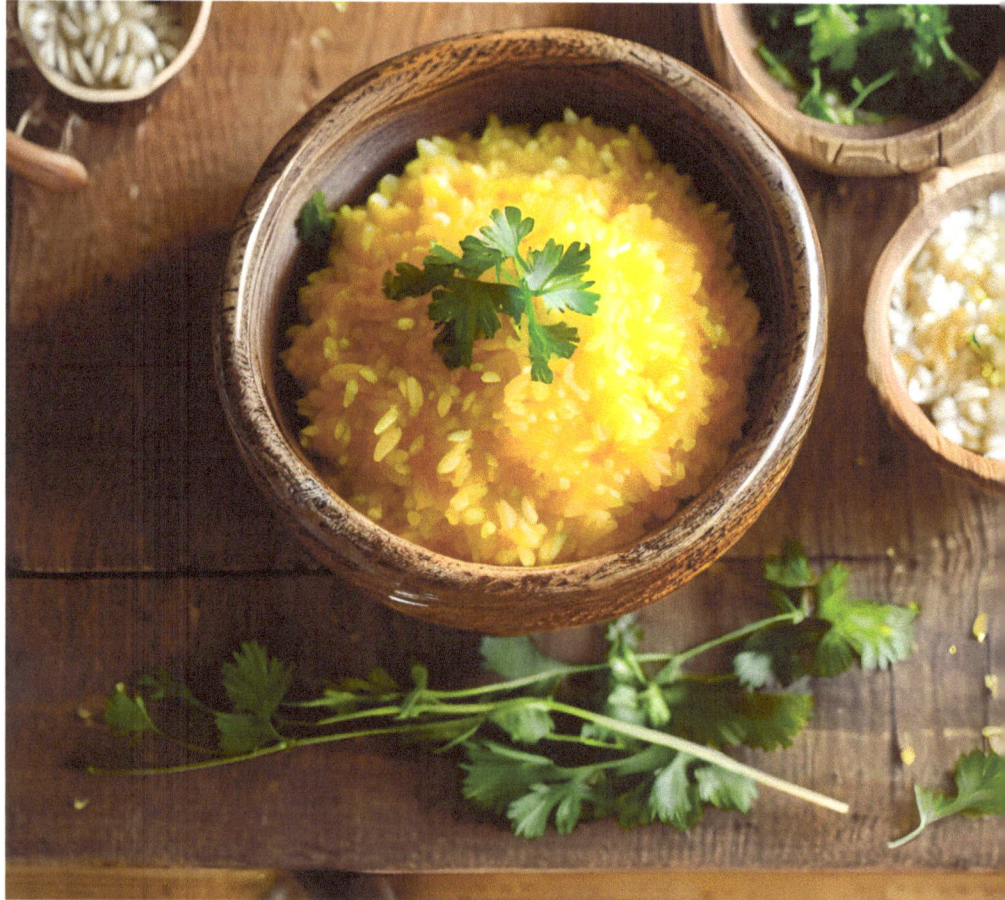

DIRECTIONS

STEP 1
Heat stock with saffron in a saucepan, keeping warm.

STEP 2
Sauté onion in butter until soft, then add rice and cook for 2 minutes.

STEP 3
Pour in white wine, allowing it to evaporate.

STEP 4
Gradually add stock, stirring continuously until rice is tender and creamy.

STEP 5
Stir in butter and Parmesan cheese before serving.

VEAL SALTIMBOCCA

Veal cutlets are paired with prosciutto and sage, then cooked in a buttery white wine sauce.

INGREDIENTS

- 4 veal cutlets
- 4 slices prosciutto
- 8 sage leaves
- 1/2 cup white wine
- 3 tbsp butter
- Salt and pepper

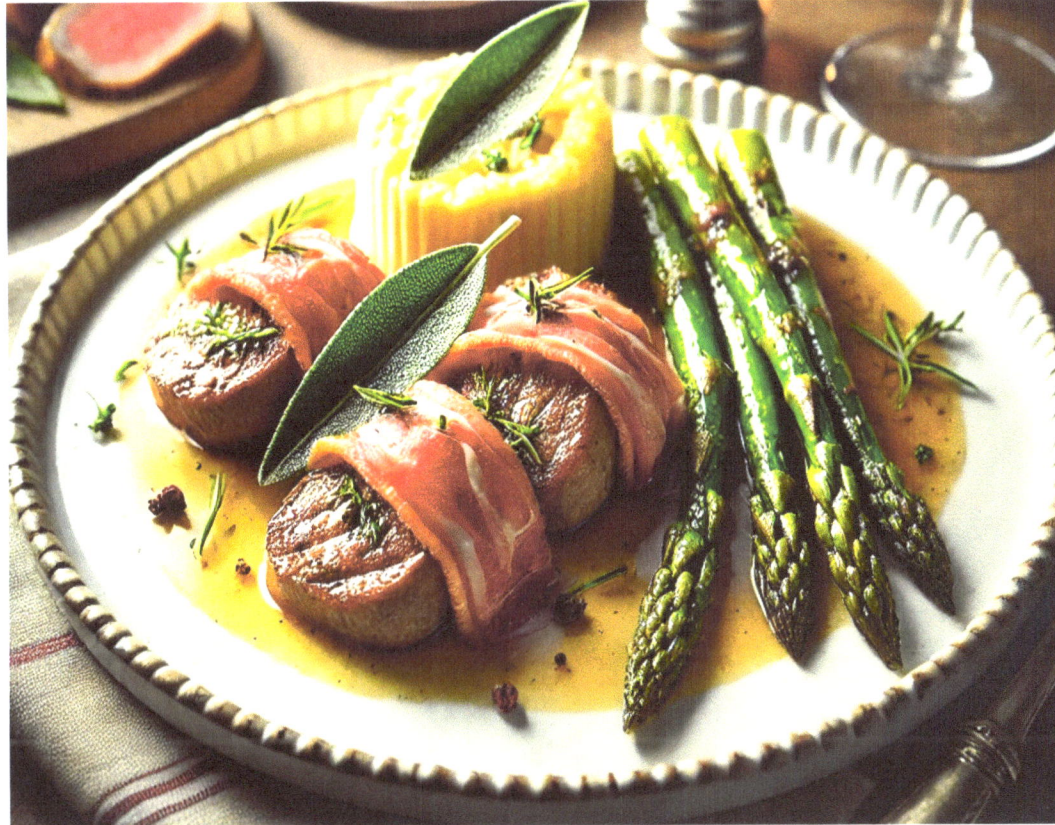

DIRECTIONS

STEP 1
Place a slice of prosciutto and two sage leaves on each veal cutlet.

STEP 2
Secure with toothpicks and sauté in butter until browned on both sides.

STEP 3
Add white wine to deglaze the pan, simmering for 5 minutes.

STEP 4
Serve with a drizzle of sauce.

PORK OSSO BUCO

A hearty pork version of the traditional osso buco, braised in a savory broth with aromatic vegetables.

INGREDIENTS

- 4 pork shanks
- 1 onion, chopped
- 2 carrots, chopped
- 2 celery stalks, chopped
- 2 garlic cloves, minced
- 1 cup white wine
- 2 cups chicken stock
- 1 tbsp tomato paste

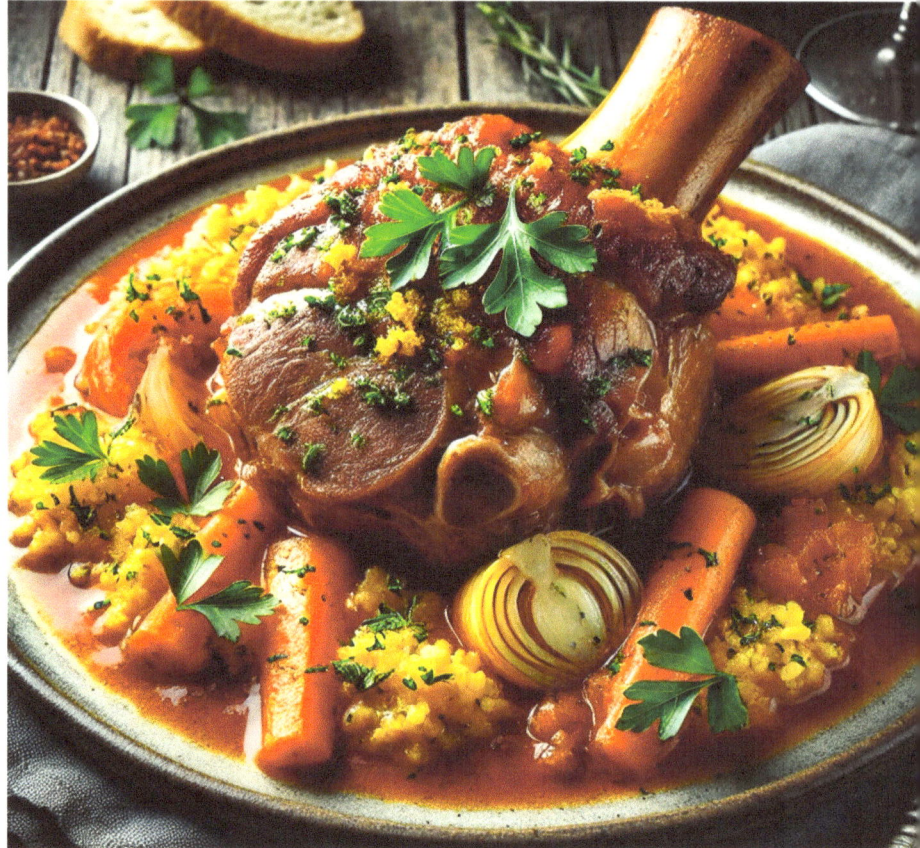

DIRECTIONS

STEP 1
Brown the pork shanks in oil and set aside.

STEP 2
Sauté onions, carrots, celery, and garlic until soft.

STEP 3
Stir in tomato paste, wine, and stock, returning pork shanks to the pot.

STEP 4
Simmer for 2 hours until meat is tender.

FRITTATA DI ZUCCHINI

A simple zucchini frittata, made with eggs, Parmesan, and fresh herbs.

INGREDIENTS

- 4 large eggs
- 2 medium zucchinis, sliced
- 1/2 cup grated Parmesan cheese
- Olive oil for frying
- Fresh basil, chopped

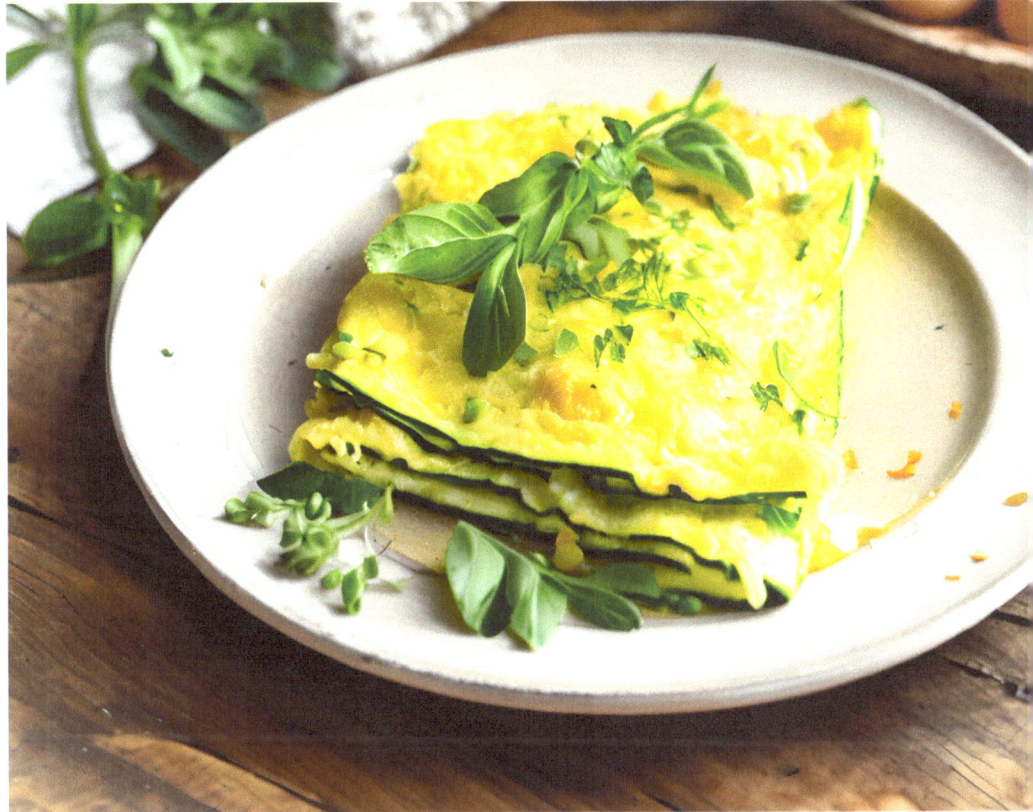

DIRECTIONS

STEP 1
Sauté zucchini in olive oil until softened.

STEP 2
Beat eggs with Parmesan and basil, then pour over zucchini.

STEP 3
Cook on low heat until eggs are set, then flip to cook the other side.

STEP 4
Serve warm.

CAPONATA

A Sicilian eggplant dish made with a mix of vegetables, olives, capers, and a sweet-and-sour vinegar sauce.

INGREDIENTS

- 2 eggplants, diced
- 1 onion, chopped
- 1 celery stalk, chopped
- 1/4 cup green olives
- 2 tbsp capers
- 1/4 cup red wine vinegar
- 2 tbsp sugar
- 1 can (14 oz) crushed tomatoes

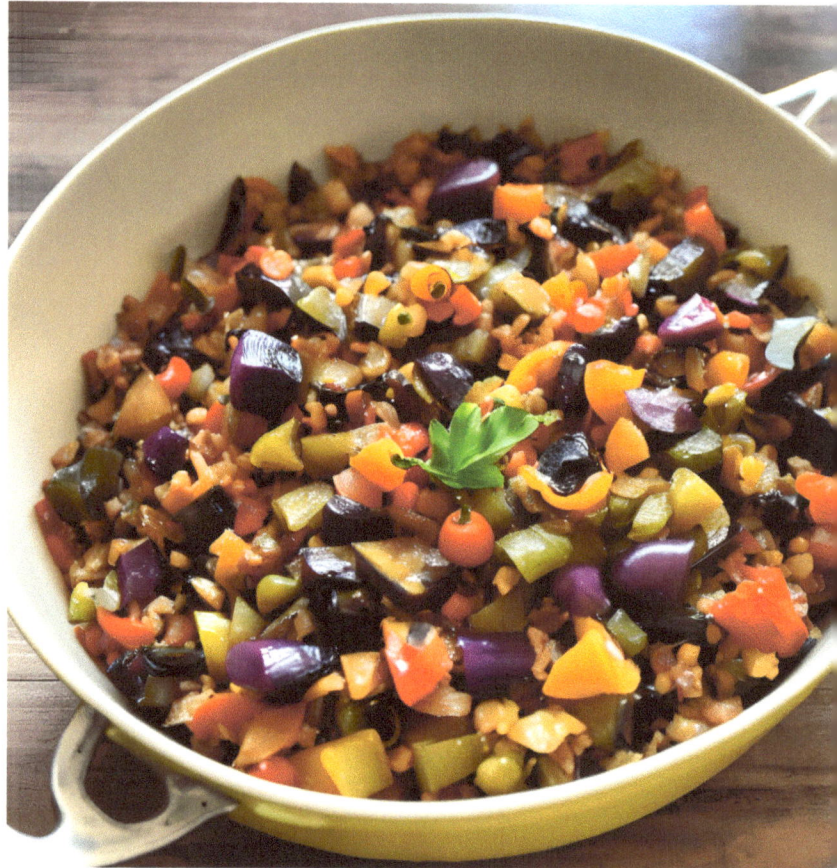

DIRECTIONS

STEP 1
Sauté eggplant in olive oil until golden, set aside.

STEP 2
In the same pan, sauté onion, celery, olives, and capers.

STEP 3
Add vinegar and sugar, simmering until syrupy.

STEP 4
Stir in tomatoes, then return eggplant to the pan and cook for 20 minutes.

STEP 5
Let cool and serve at room temperature.

POLLO ALLA CACCIATORA

Chicken cooked in a tomato sauce with olives, capers, and herbs, resulting in a robust, flavorful dish.

INGREDIENTS

- 4 chicken thighs
- 1 can (14 oz) diced tomatoes
- 1/4 cup black olives
- 2 tbsp capers
- 1 onion, chopped
- 2 garlic cloves, minced
- 1/4 cup red wine
- Fresh rosemary

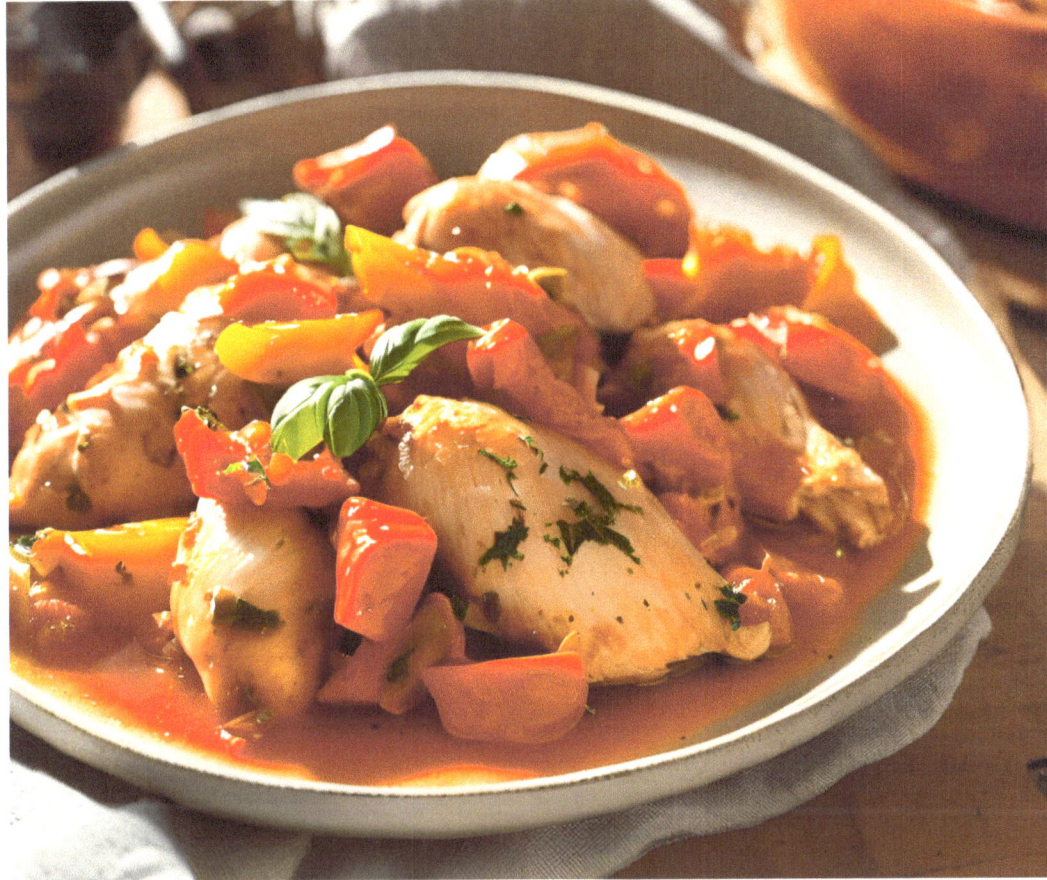

DIRECTIONS

STEP 1
Brown the chicken thighs in a pan and set aside.

STEP 2
Sauté onions and garlic in olive oil, then add tomatoes, olives, capers, and red wine.

STEP 3
Return chicken to the pan, simmering for 40 minutes.

STEP 4
Garnish with rosemary before serving.

PASTA ALLA NORMA

This iconic Sicilian dish combines fried eggplant, tomato sauce, and ricotta salata, creating a perfect balance of savory flavors.

INGREDIENTS

- 1 lb pasta (penne or rigatoni)
- 2 medium eggplants, diced
- 1 can (14 oz) crushed tomatoes
- 1/4 cup fresh basil
- 1/4 cup ricotta salata, grated
- Olive oil for frying

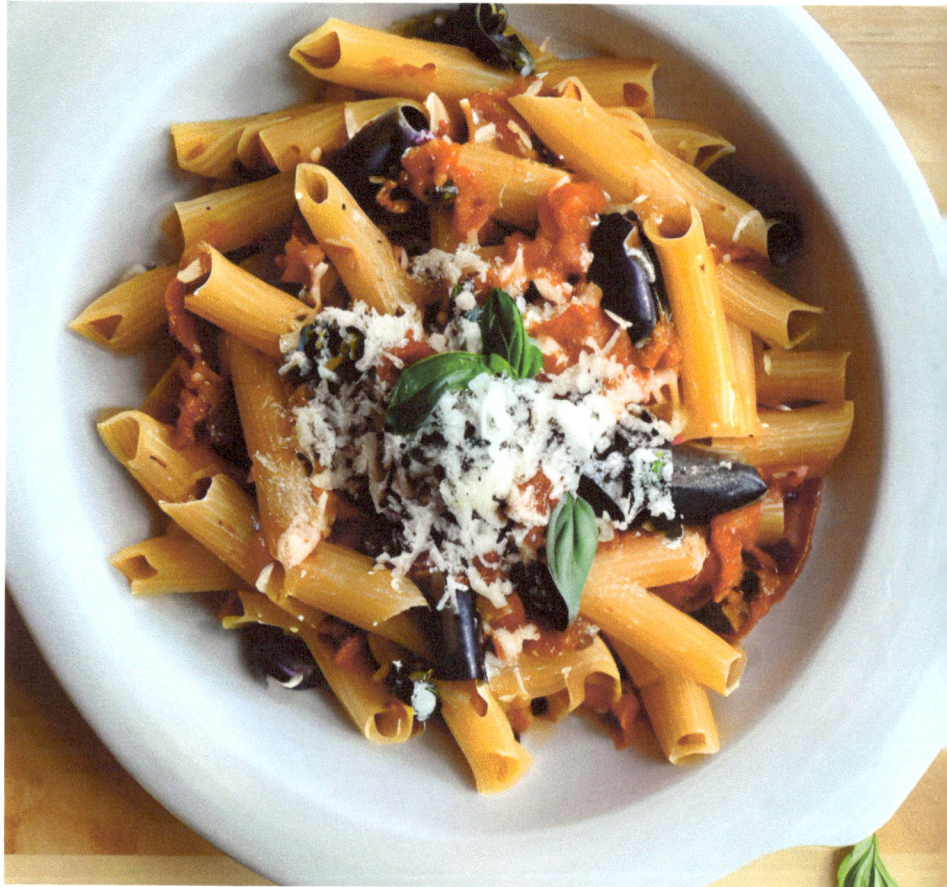

DIRECTIONS

STEP 1
Fry the diced eggplant in olive oil until golden, then drain on paper towels.

STEP 2
Prepare pasta according to package instructions.

STEP 3
Simmer crushed tomatoes with garlic and basil in a pan.

STEP 4
Toss cooked pasta with tomato sauce, fried eggplant, and grated ricotta salata.

STEP 5
Serve garnished with fresh basil.

PORCHETTA

A succulent, slow-roasted pork dish, seasoned with garlic, rosemary, and fennel, often served as a main course for celebrations.

INGREDIENTS

- 3-4 lb boneless pork belly
- 4 cloves garlic, minced
- 2 tbsp fresh rosemary, chopped
- 2 tbsp fennel seeds
- 1/4 cup white wine
- Olive oil

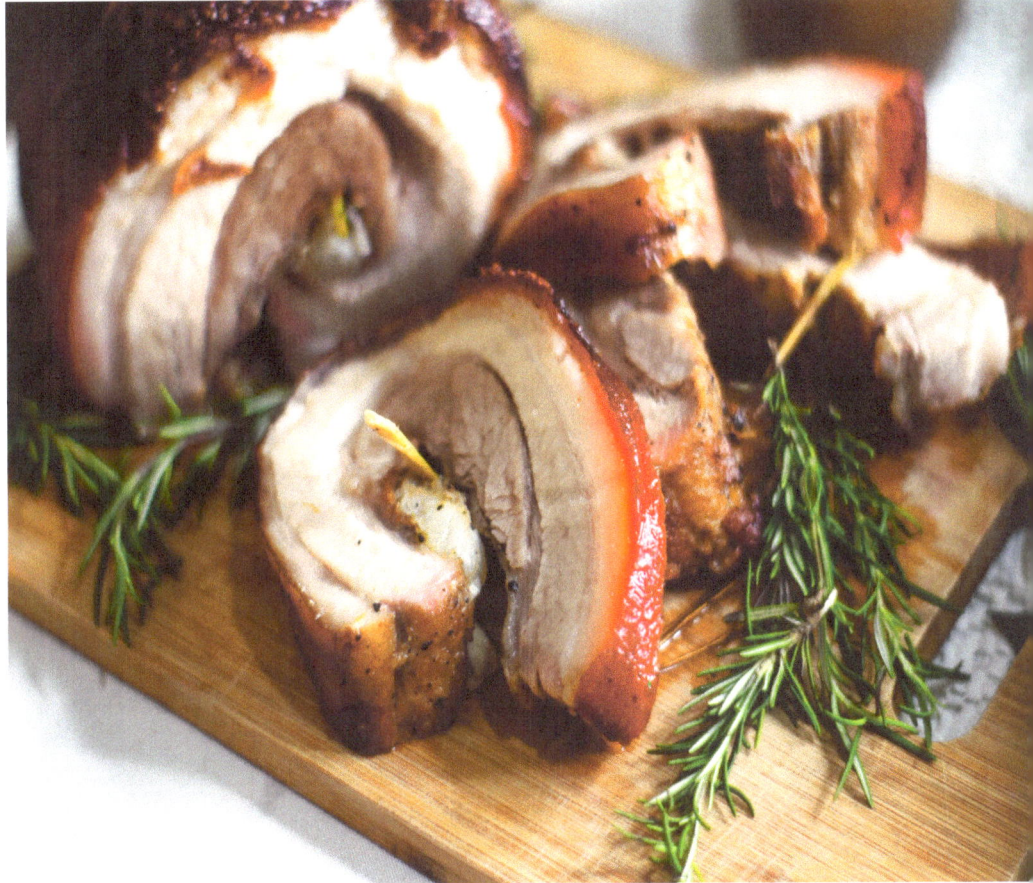

DIRECTIONS

STEP 1

Butterfly the pork belly and season with garlic, rosemary, fennel seeds, salt, and pepper.

STEP 2

Roll the pork, tie it with twine, and roast at 375°F for about 2 hours, basting occasionally with white wine and olive oil.

STEP 3

Let rest for 10 minutes before slicing and serving.

FRITTURA DI PESCE
(MIXED FRIED FISH)

A classic Italian seafood dish featuring a variety of fish and shellfish, lightly battered and deep-fried.

INGREDIENTS

- 1 lb mixed seafood (squid, shrimp, small fish fillets)
- 1 cup all-purpose flour
- 1 egg, beaten
- Olive oil for frying
- Lemon wedges

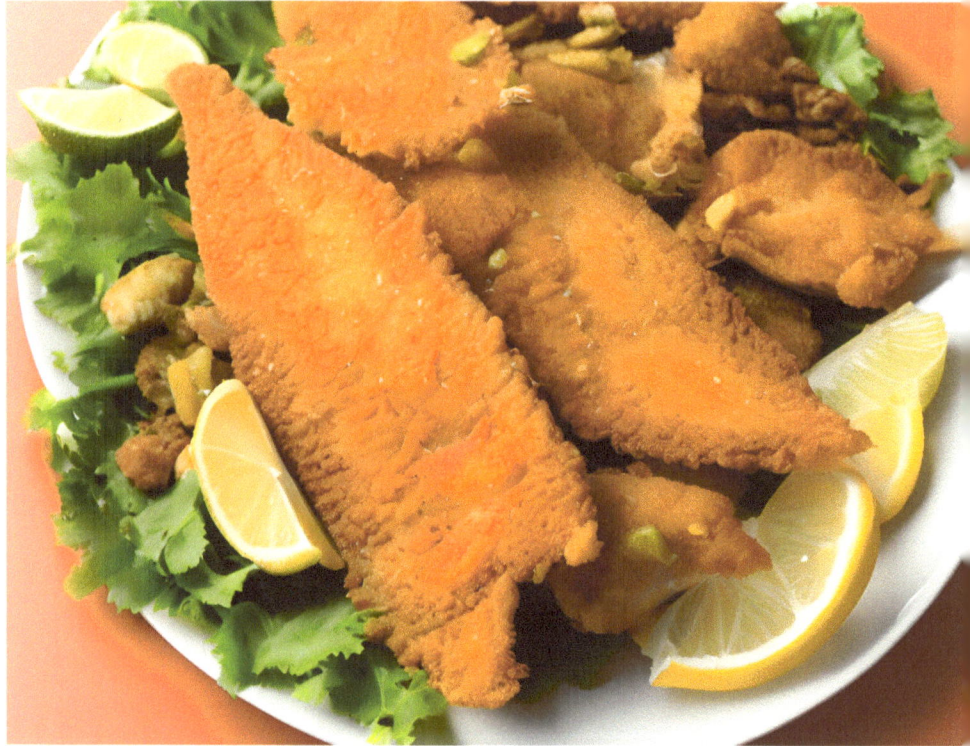

DIRECTIONS

STEP 1
Heat oil in a deep fryer or pan.

STEP 2
Dip seafood in beaten egg, then dredge in flour.

STEP 3
Fry in batches until golden brown, about 3-4 minutes.

STEP 4
Drain on paper towels and serve with lemon wedges.

RISOTTO AI FUNGHI
(MUSHROOM RISOTTO)

A creamy, savory risotto with earthy mushrooms and a touch of Parmesan, perfect as an entrée or side dish.

INGREDIENTS

- 1 1/2 cups Arborio rice
- 4 cups vegetable or chicken broth
- 1 lb mixed mushrooms (porcini, cremini, etc.), sliced
- 1/2 cup dry white wine
- 1/4 cup grated Parmesan cheese
- 2 tbsp butter

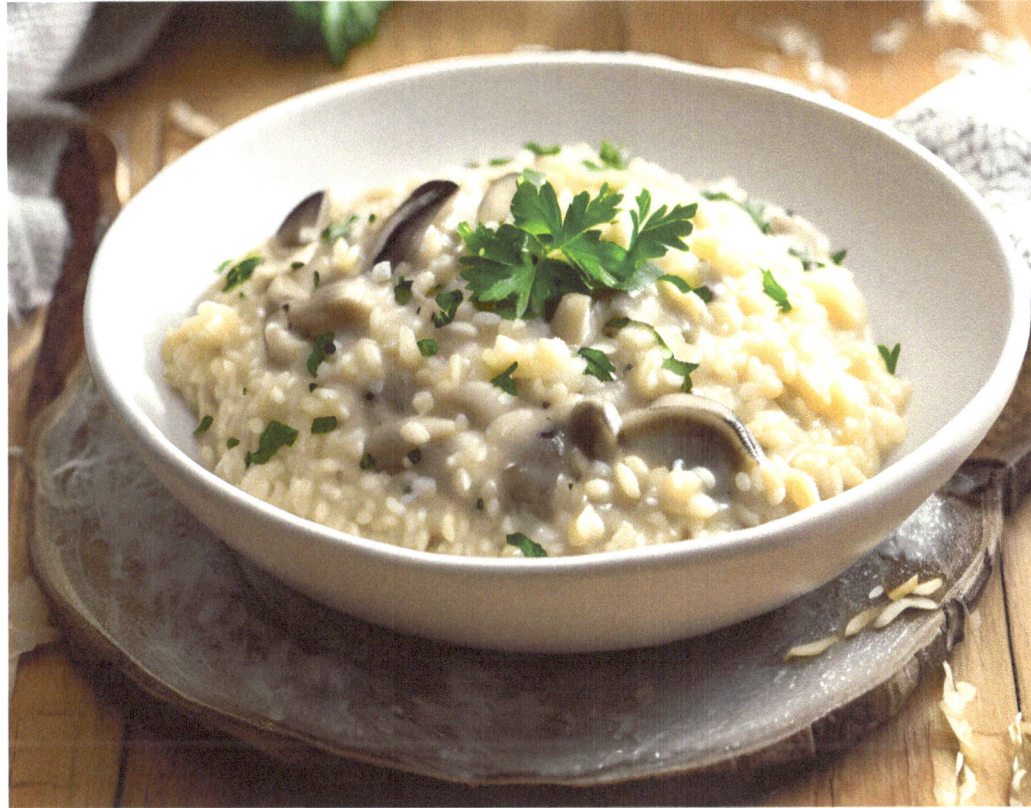

DIRECTIONS

STEP 1

Sauté mushrooms in butter until softened and set aside.

STEP 2

In the same pan, toast Arborio rice until lightly golden.

STEP 3

Gradually add warm broth, stirring constantly until rice is cooked and creamy.

STEP 4

Stir in mushrooms, wine, and Parmesan cheese, then cook for a few more minutes.

SALSICCIA E FAGIOLI (SAUSAGE AND BEANS)

A hearty dish made with Italian sausage, cannellini beans, and a tomato-based sauce, perfect for cooler weather.

INGREDIENTS

- 4 Italian sausages (mild or spicy)
- 2 cans (14 oz each) cannellini beans, drained
- 1 can (14 oz) diced tomatoes
- 1 onion, chopped
- 2 garlic cloves, minced
- Olive oil

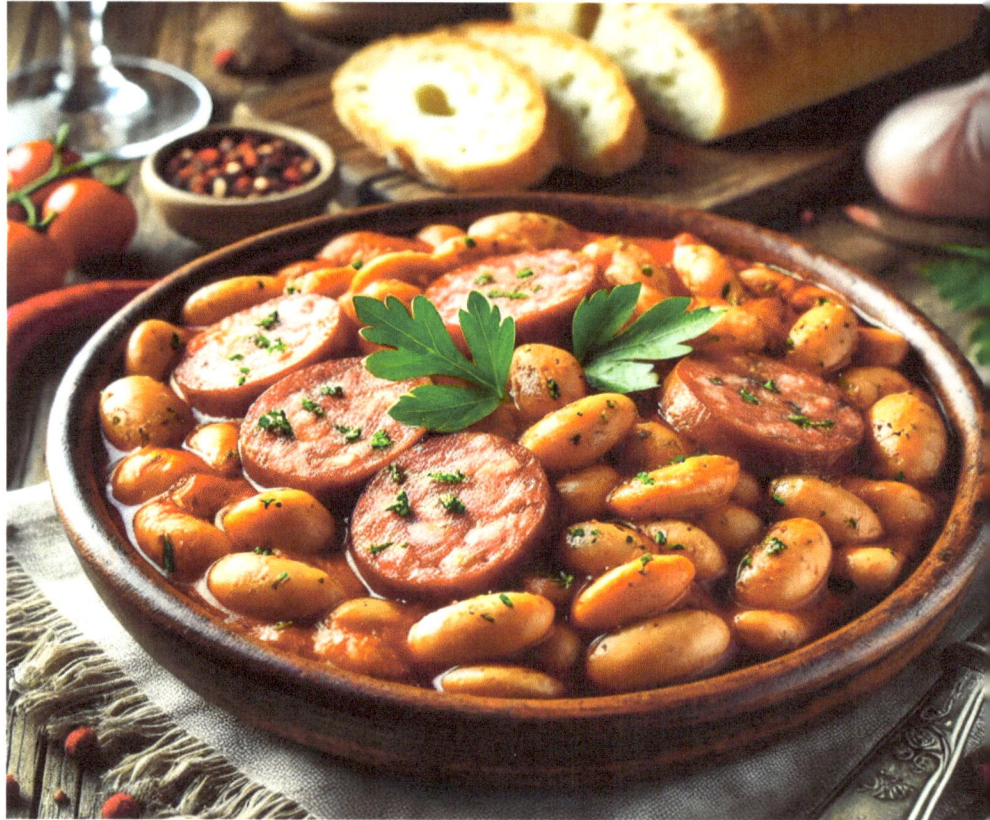

DIRECTIONS

STEP 1
Brown sausages in a skillet, then set aside.

STEP 2
In the same pan, sauté onions and garlic until softened.

STEP 3
Add beans, tomatoes, and sausages back into the pan, simmering for 20-30 minutes.

STEP 4
Serve with crusty bread.

TAGLIATA DI MANZO

A Tuscan-style steak, typically grilled and served sliced thinly, with a drizzle of olive oil and a sprinkle of arugula.

INGREDIENTS

- 2 ribeye steaks
- Olive oil
- Fresh arugula
- Sea salt and black pepper
- Balsamic vinegar (optional)

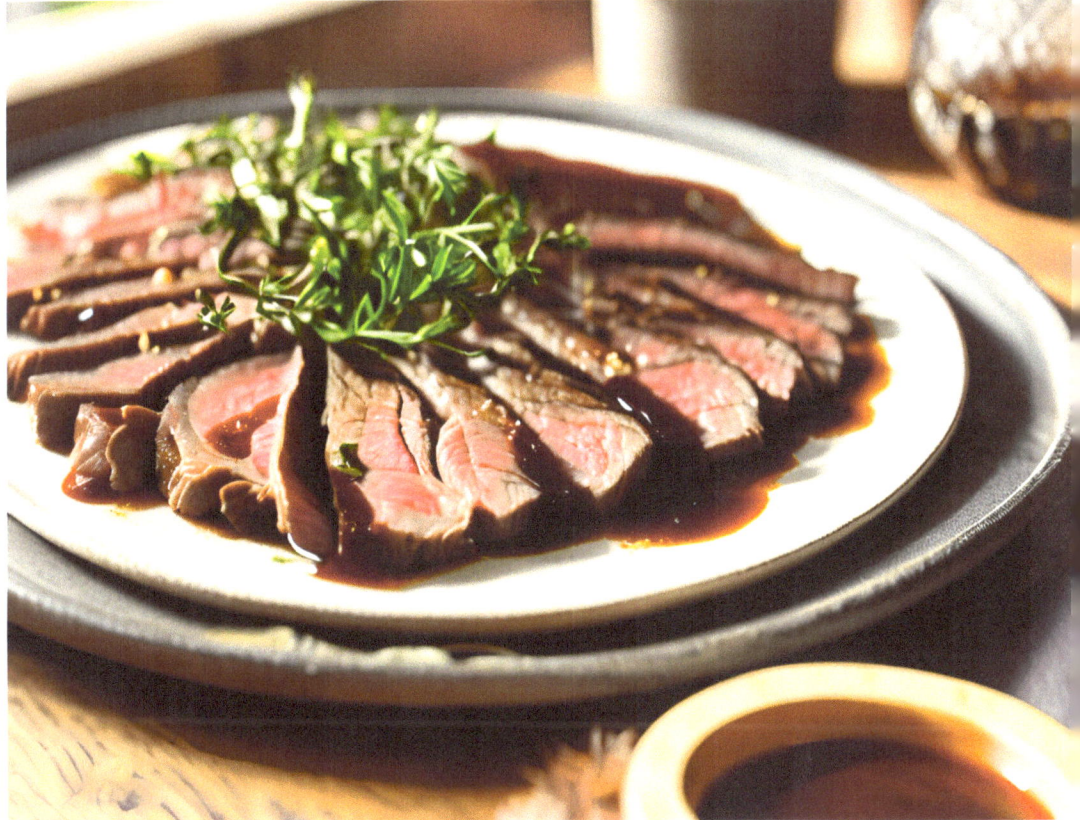

DIRECTIONS

STEP 1

Grill steaks to desired doneness.

STEP 2

Let rest for 5 minutes before slicing thinly against the grain.

STEP 3

Arrange on a platter with fresh arugula, drizzle with olive oil, and season with salt and pepper. Optional: Drizzle with balsamic vinegar.

POLENTA CON FUNGHI
(POLENTA WITH MUSHROOMS)

Creamy polenta topped with sautéed mushrooms, a classic dish from northern Italy.

INGREDIENTS

- 1 cup cornmeal
- 4 cups water
- 2 tbsp butter
- 1 lb mixed mushrooms, sliced
- 1/2 cup Parmesan cheese

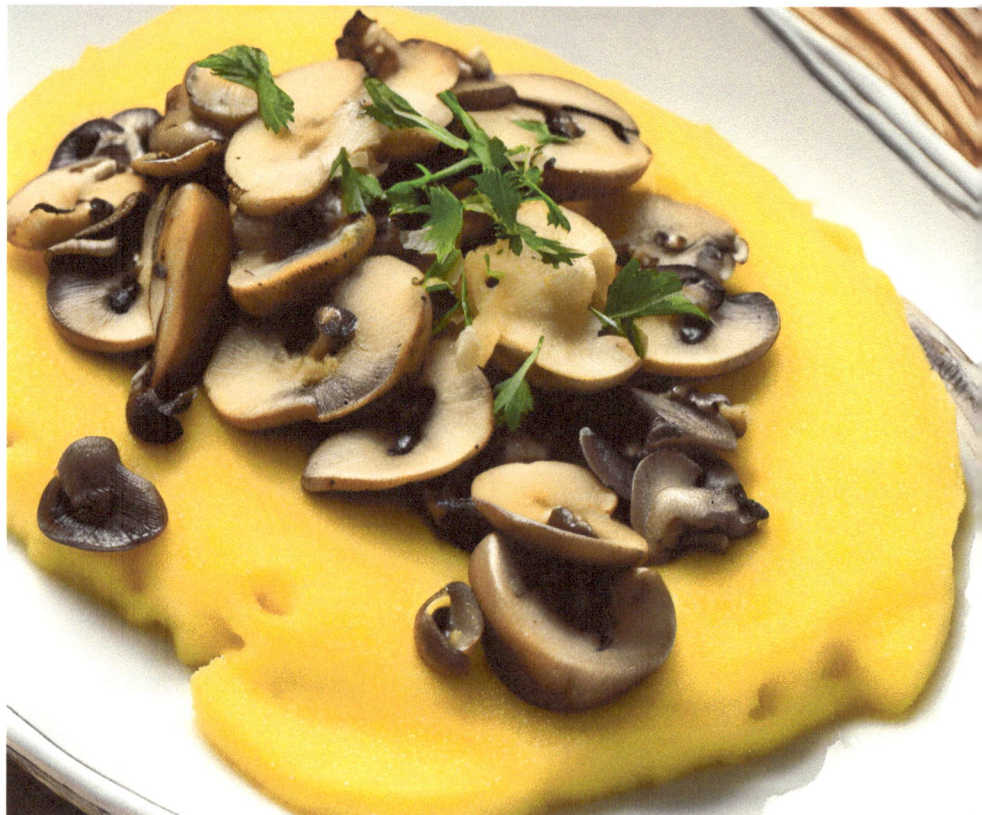

DIRECTIONS

STEP 1
Cook cornmeal in boiling water, stirring frequently until thick and creamy.

STEP 2
Sauté mushrooms in butter until tender.

STEP 3
Serve polenta topped with sautéed mushrooms and Parmesan cheese.

TORTELLINI EN BRODO

Small stuffed pasta served in a rich broth, perfect as a comforting winter dish.

- 1 lb fresh tortellini (cheese or meat-filled)
- 4 cups chicken or beef broth
- 1 tbsp fresh parsley, chopped
- Fresh Parmesan cheese, grated

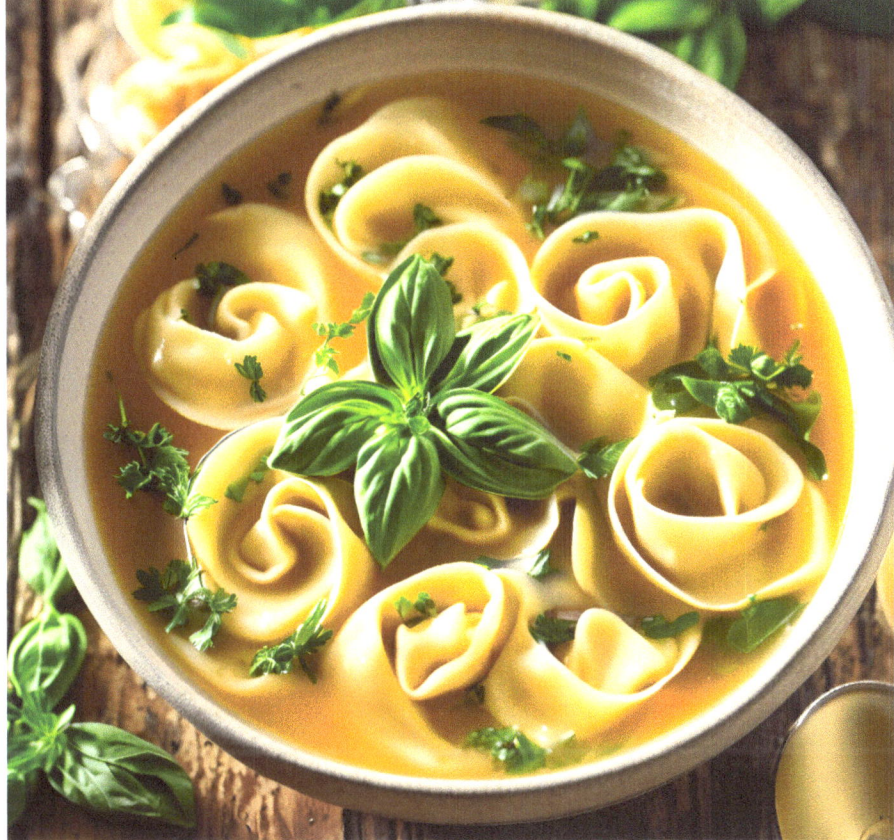

DIRECTIONS

STEP 1

Bring the broth to a simmer.

STEP 2

Cook tortellini according to package instructions, then add to the broth.

STEP 3

Serve with fresh parsley and grated Parmesan cheese.

POLLO AL LIMONE

A simple yet flavorful dish where chicken is sautéed with lemon, garlic, and white wine, making it a bright, tangy entrée.

INGREDIENTS

- 4 boneless chicken breasts
- 2 lemons (zested and juiced)
- 1/2 cup white wine
- 3 tbsp olive oil
- 2 garlic cloves, minced

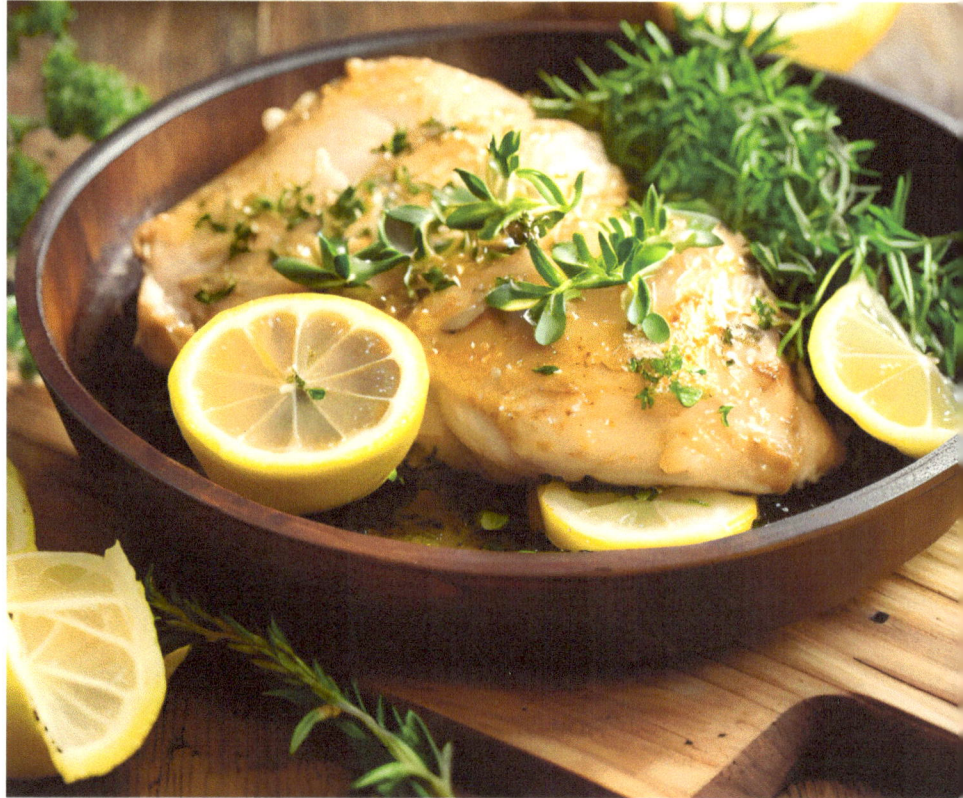

DIRECTIONS

STEP 1

Sauté chicken in olive oil until golden and cooked through.

STEP 2

Remove chicken and deglaze the pan with white wine, adding lemon juice, zest, and garlic.

STEP 3

Return chicken to the pan, simmering for 5 minutes to allow flavors to meld.

COTOLETTE ALLA MILANESE

A breaded and fried veal or pork cutlet, similar to a schnitzel, that is crispy on the outside and tender on the inside.

- 4 veal or pork cutlets
- 2 eggs, beaten
- 1 1/2 cups breadcrumbs
- Olive oil for frying
- Lemon wedges

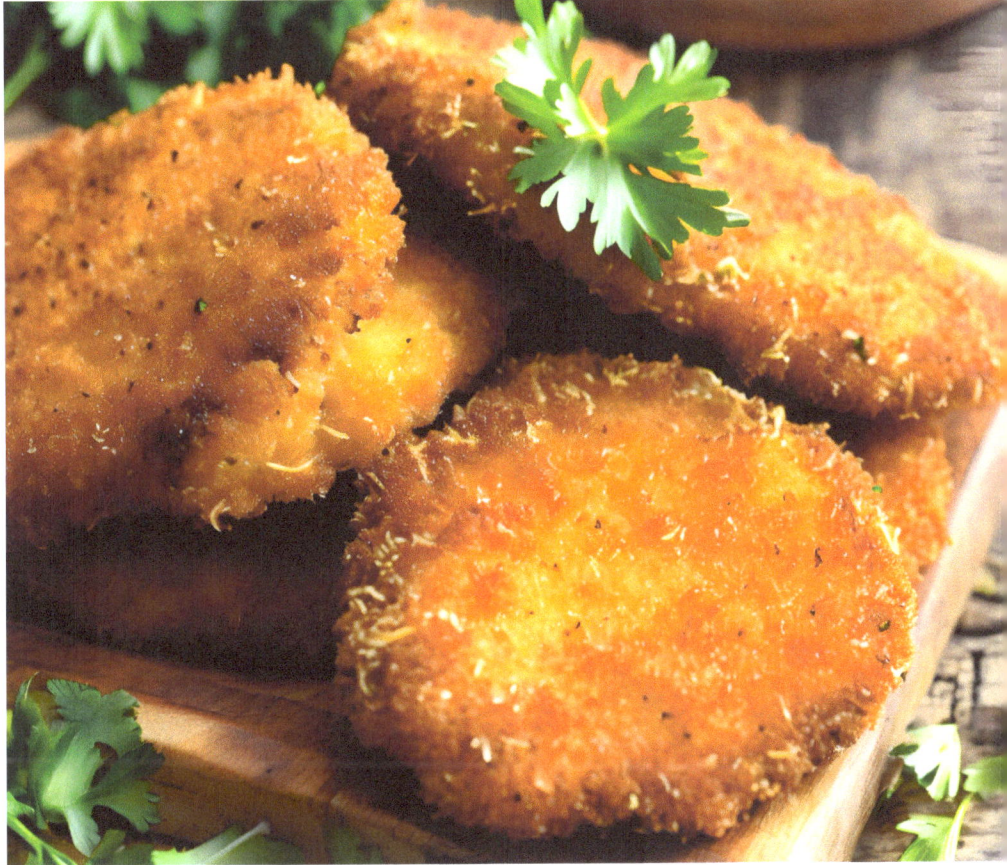

DIRECTIONS

STEP 1

Dredge cutlets in flour, dip in beaten eggs, and coat with breadcrumbs.

STEP 2

Fry in hot oil until golden brown on both sides, about 3-4 minutes per side.

STEP 3

Serve with a squeeze of lemon.

CAPONATA SICILIANA

A sweet and sour eggplant dish from Sicily, featuring a medley of vegetables, olives, capers, and a tangy tomato sauce.

INGREDIENTS

- 2 large eggplants, diced
- 1 onion, chopped
- 1 cup green olives, pitted
- 1/4 cup capers
- 2 tbsp red wine vinegar
- 1 can (14 oz) diced tomatoes
- 1 tbsp sugar
- Olive oil for frying

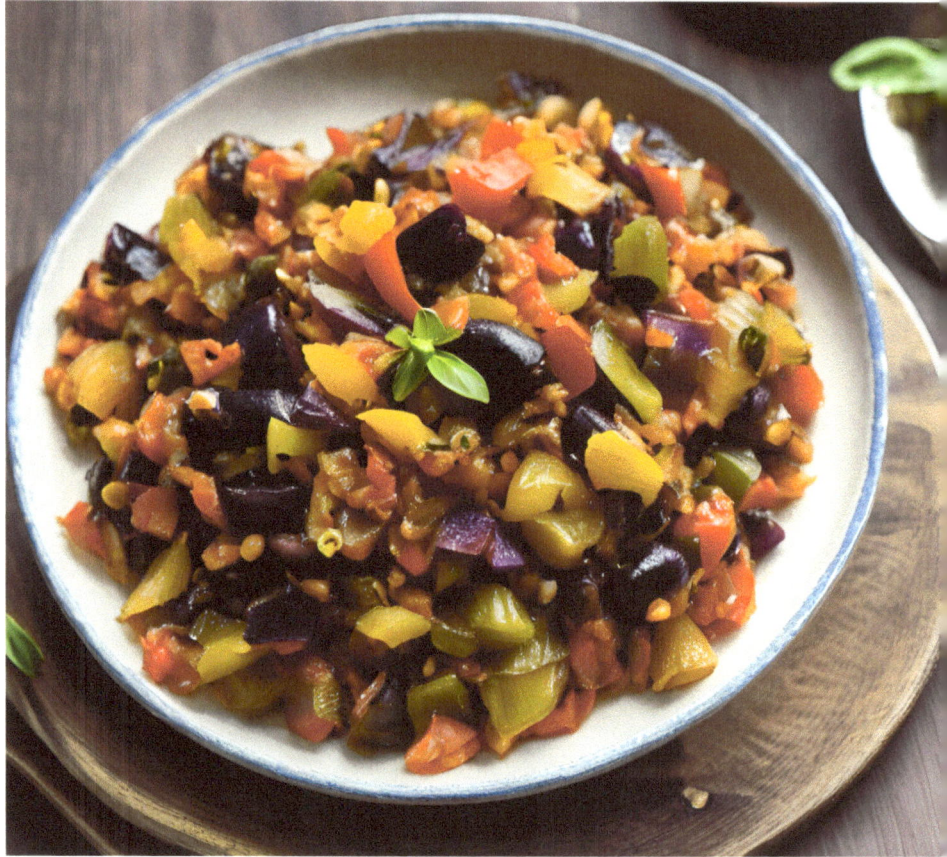

DIRECTIONS

STEP 1
Fry eggplant cubes in olive oil until golden, then drain on paper towels.

STEP 2
In the same pan, sauté onions, olives, and capers.

STEP 3
Add tomatoes, vinegar, and sugar, simmering for 10 minutes.

STEP 4
Add the fried eggplant to the pan and cook for another 5 minutes.

STEP 5
Serve warm or at room temperature.

ARISTA DI MAIALE
(TUSCAN ROAST PORK)

A traditional Tuscan dish, this roast pork is seasoned with garlic, rosemary, and olive oil, and slow-roasted until golden and tender.

INGREDIENTS

- 4 lb boneless pork loin
- 4 garlic cloves, minced
- 3 sprigs fresh rosemary
- 1/4 cup olive oil
- 1 cup white wine

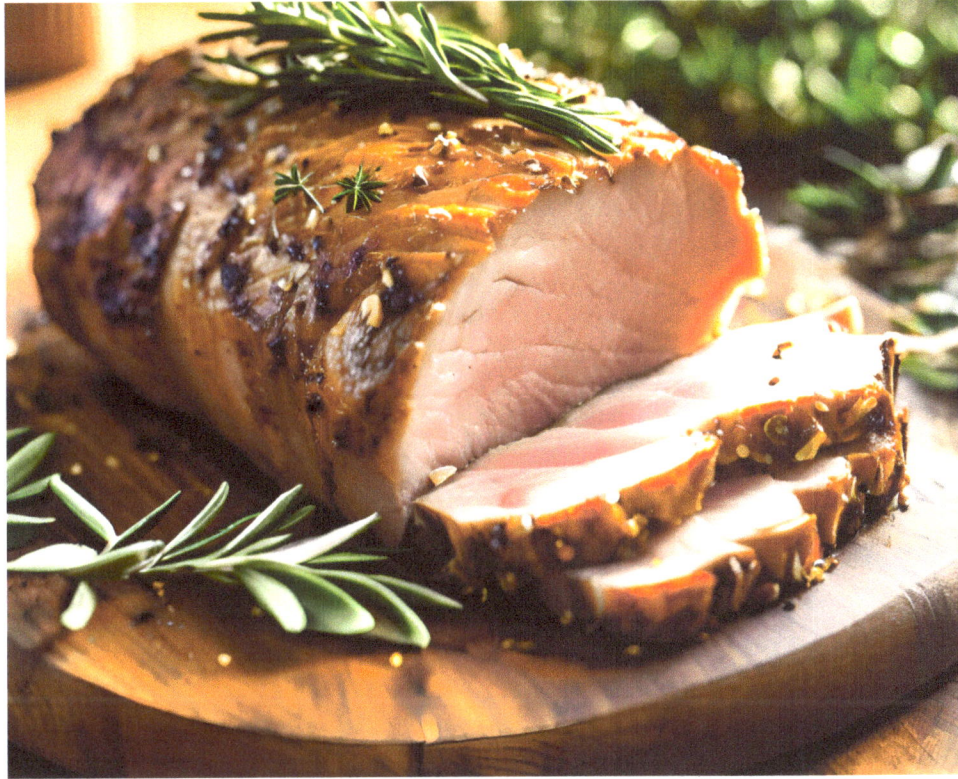

DIRECTIONS

STEP 1
Preheat oven to 375°F. Rub the pork with garlic, rosemary, salt, and pepper.

STEP 2
Heat olive oil in a roasting pan, then sear the pork on all sides until browned.

STEP 3
Add white wine to the pan and roast in the oven for about 1.5 to 2 hours, basting occasionally with the pan juices.

STEP 4
Let rest for 10 minutes before slicing.

PAPPARDELLE AL BRAISED SHORT RIB RAGU

A hearty and flavorful pasta dish, where pappardelle pasta is paired with a rich wild boar ragu.

INGREDIENTS

- 1 lb pappardelle pasta
- 2 lb boneless short rib
- 1 onion, chopped
- 2 carrots, chopped
- 2 celery stalks, chopped
- 1/2 cup red wine
- 2 cups beef broth
- 1 tbsp tomato paste
- Olive oil for sautéing

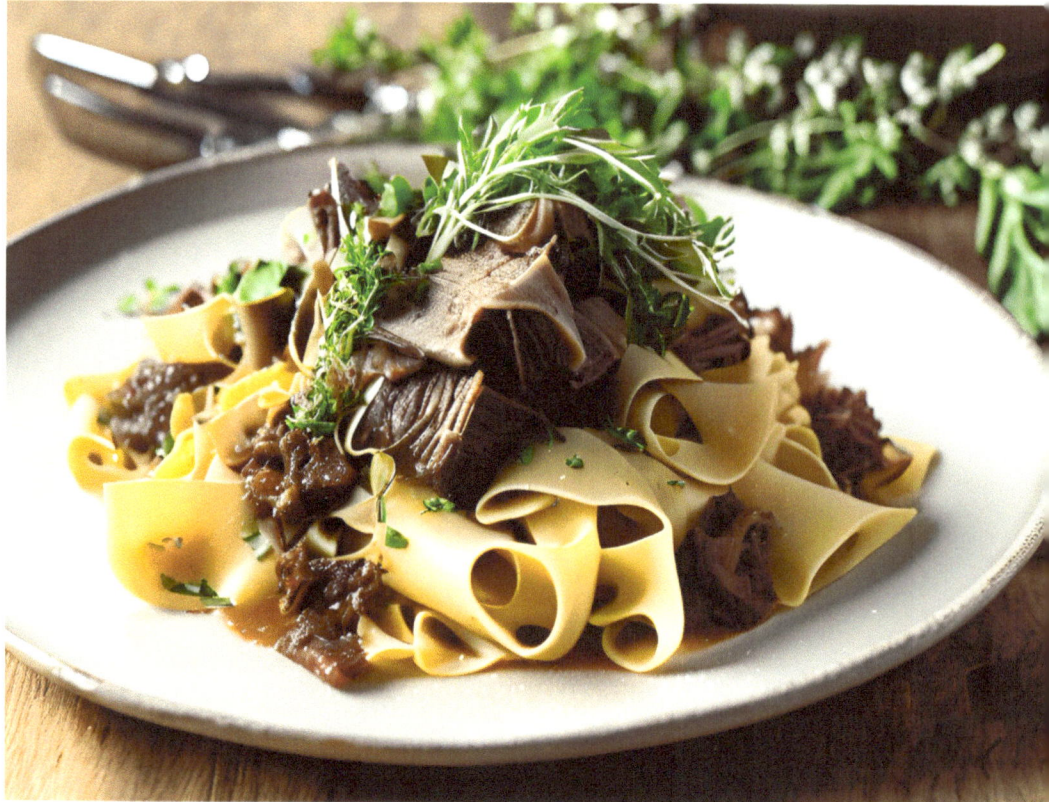

DIRECTIONS

STEP 1
Brown short ribs in olive oil, then remove and set aside.

STEP 2
Sauté onions, carrots, and celery in the same pan until soft.

STEP 3
Add tomato paste and red wine, simmering for a few minutes.

STEP 4
Return the meat to the pan, add beef broth, and simmer for 2 hours until the meat is tender.

STEP 5
Cook pappardelle according to package directions, then toss with the wild short rib ragu..

FAGOTTINI DI PROSCIUTTO E FORMAGGIO

These are delightful little bundles of prosciutto and cheese wrapped in puff pastry, baked until golden.

INGREDIENTS

- 8 slices prosciutto
- 8 oz mozzarella cheese, sliced
- 1 sheet puff pastry
- 1 egg, beaten

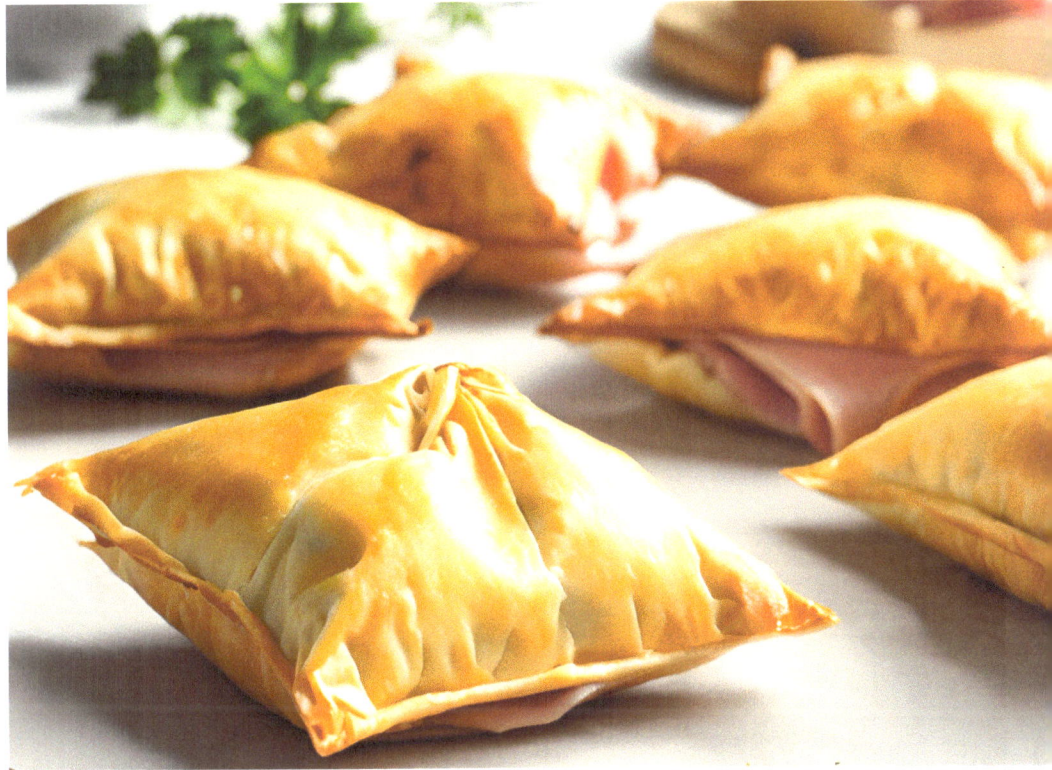

DIRECTIONS

STEP 1

Preheat oven to 375°F.

STEP 2

Place a slice of prosciutto on each square of puff pastry, followed by a slice of mozzarella.

STEP 3

Fold the pastry into a bundle and seal the edges.

STEP 4

Brush the bundles with beaten egg and bake for 20-25 minutes until golden and puffed.

VEAL FRANCAISE RECIPE

Serves: 4   Prep Time: 15 minutes   Cook Time: 20 minutes   Total Time: 35 minutes

INGREDIENTS

For the Veal
- 1 lb veal cutlets (about 8 thin pieces)
- Salt and black pepper, to taste
- 1 cup all-purpose flour
- 3 large eggs
- 2 tablespoons milk
- 3 tablespoons unsalted butter
- 2 tablespoons olive oil

For the Sauce
- 1/2 cup dry white wine
- 1/2 cup chicken stock
- 1/4 cup freshly squeezed lemon juice (about 1–2 lemons)
- 3 tablespoons unsalted butter
- 2 tablespoons fresh parsley, chopped
- Lemon slices, for garnish (optional)

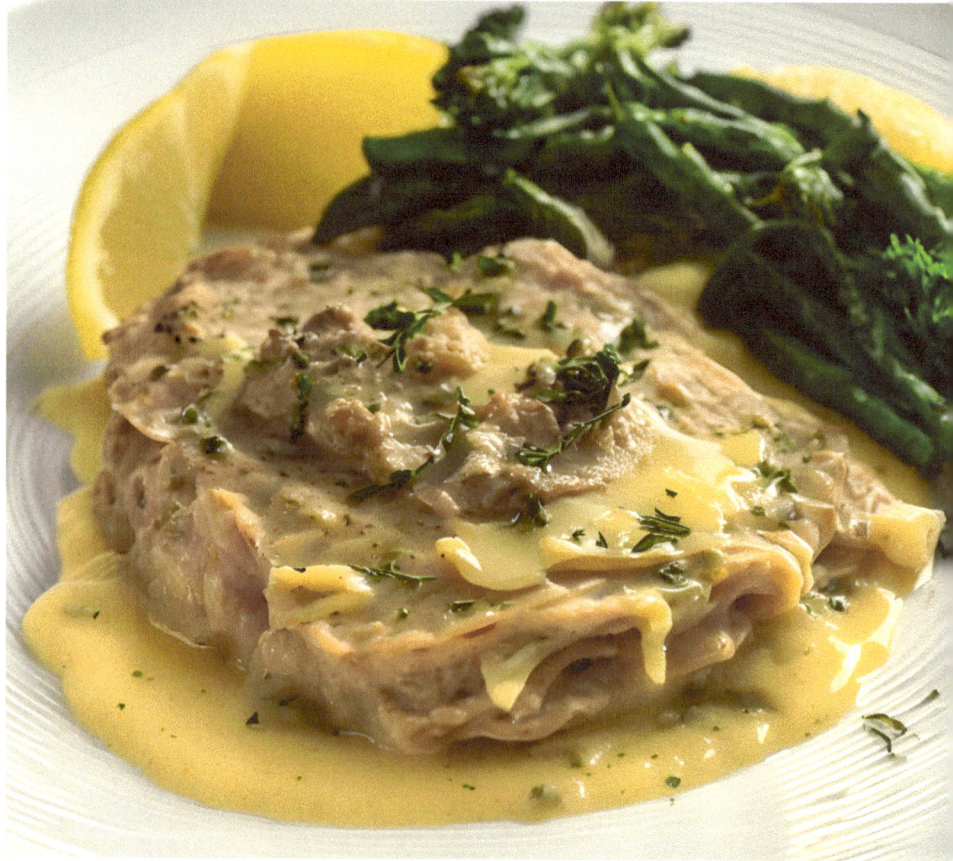

INSTRUCTIONS

Season the veal cutlets with salt and pepper on both sides. Place the flour in a shallow dish, and in another shallow dish, whisk together the eggs and milk until well blended.

Dredge each veal cutlet in the flour, shaking off any excess. Then dip each floured cutlet into the egg mixture, ensuring it's fully coated. Heat a large skillet over medium heat and add 2 tablespoons of butter and 2 tablespoons of olive oil. Once the butter has melted and is sizzling, add the veal cutlets in batches to avoid overcrowding. Cook each cutlet for 2–3 minutes on each side, until golden brown. Transfer the cooked veal to a plate and set aside, repeating with remaining cutlets and adding more butter or oil if needed.

In the same skillet, add the white wine, stirring to deglaze the pan and loosen any browned bits. Add the chicken stock and lemon juice, stirring well. Let the sauce simmer for 3–4 minutes, reducing slightly.

Lower the heat and add 3 tablespoons of butter to the skillet, stirring constantly until it melts and the sauce thickens slightly. Add the fresh parsley, then return the veal cutlets to the skillet, spooning the sauce over each piece.

Arrange the veal cutlets on a serving platter, pouring the remaining sauce over the top. Garnish with lemon slices and extra parsley if desired.

BACCALÀ ALLA VICENTINA (SALTED COD VICENTINA STYLE)

A Veneto region specialty, this dish features salted cod slowly stewed with onions, anchovies, and milk.

INGREDIENTS

- 1 lb salted cod, soaked overnight
- 2 onions, chopped
- 2 anchovy fillets
- 1 cup whole milk
- Olive oil for frying

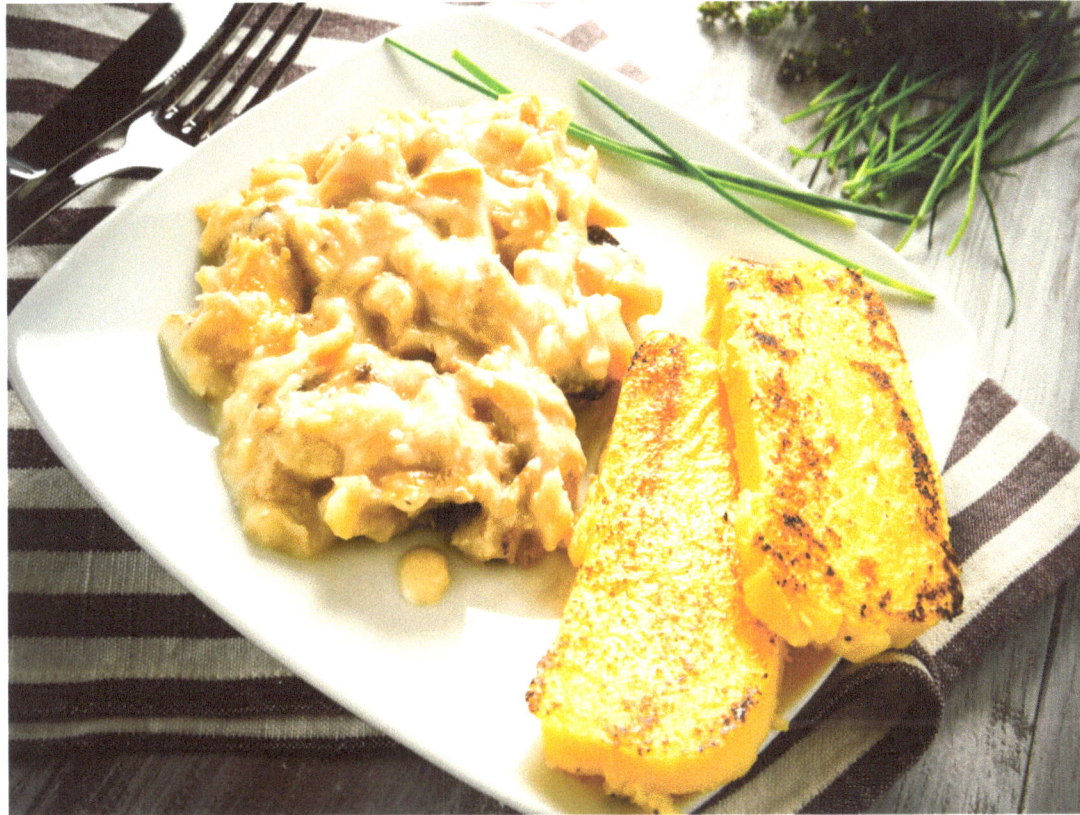

DIRECTIONS

STEP 1

Sauté onions and anchovies in olive oil until softened.

STEP 2

Add soaked cod and milk, cooking on low for 2 hours, stirring occasionally.

STEP 3

Serve with polenta for a traditional pairing.

ZUCCHINI LASAGANA ALLA BOLOGNESE

A traditional Italian lasagna made with layers of rich Bolognese sauce, béchamel, and pasta.

INGREDIENTS

- 1 lb ground beef
- 1 onion, chopped
- 4 cups tomato sauce
- Two whole zucchini
- 2 cups ricotta cheese
- ¼ cup parm cheese
- ½ cup shredded mozzerella
- 1 whole egg

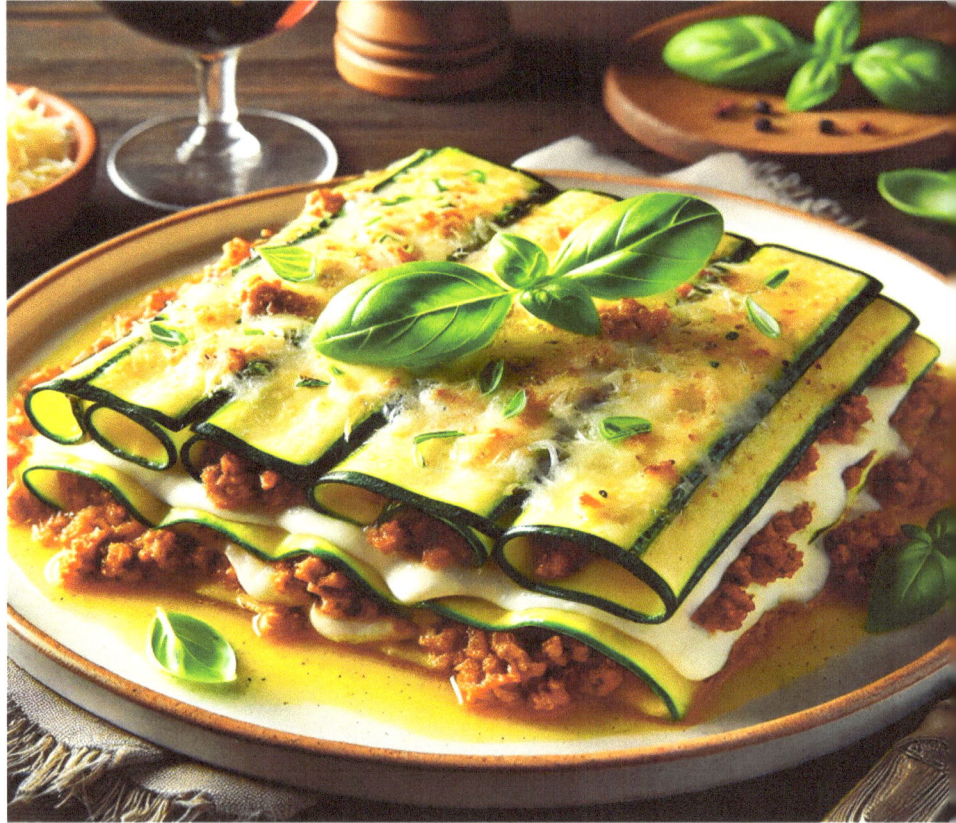

DIRECTIONS

STEP 1

Brown ground beef with onion, then add tomato sauce and simmer for 1 hour.

STEP 2

Mix Bolognese with ricotta, egg, and parmesan

STEP 3

Slice zucchini lengthwise on the mandolin-lay in colander with salt, pat dry

STEP 4

In pan layer sauce, zucchini, bolognese, mozzarella, repeat

STEP 5

Top with Bolognese and mozzerella

STEP 6

Bake at 375°F for 45 minutes, then let rest before serving.

SPAGHETTI ALLE VONGOLE
(SPAGHETTI WITH CLAMS)

A simple yet elegant seafood pasta dish made with fresh clams, garlic, white wine, and parsley.

INGREDIENTS

- 1 lb spaghetti
- 2 lbs fresh clams, cleaned
- 4 garlic cloves, minced
- 1/2 cup dry white wine
- 1/4 cup fresh parsley, chopped
- Olive oil for sautéing

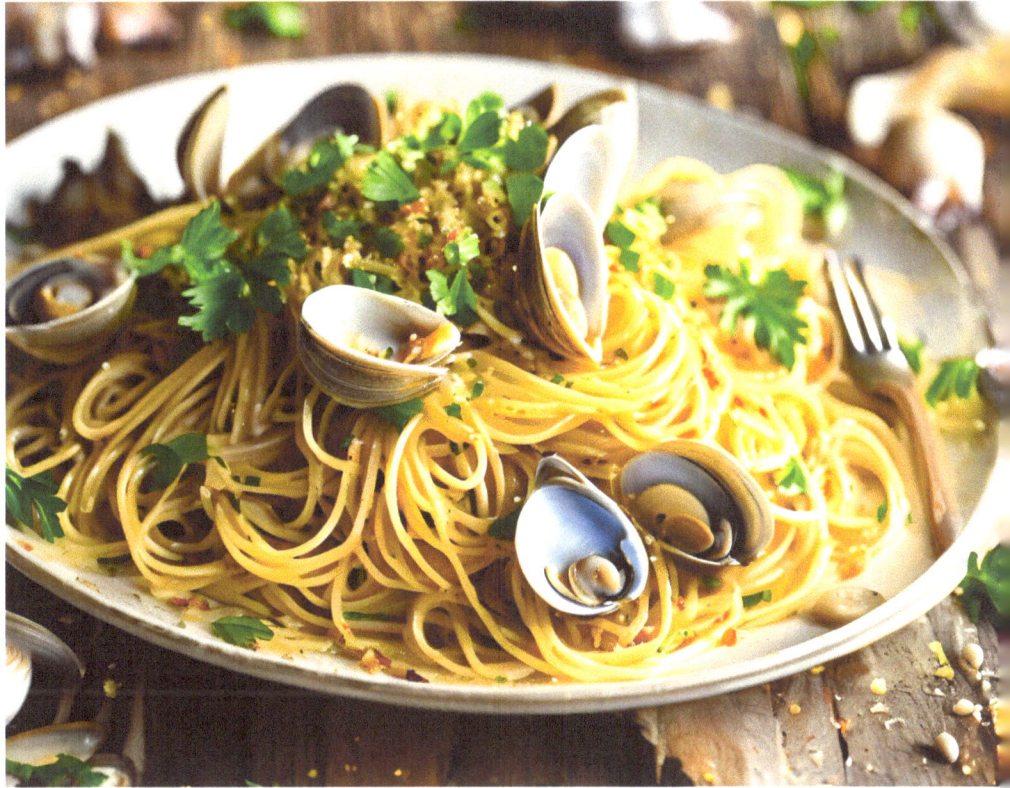

DIRECTIONS

STEP 1

Cook spaghetti according to package instructions.

STEP 2

Sauté garlic in olive oil until fragrant, then add clams and white wine.

STEP 3

Cover and cook until clams open, then toss with spaghetti and fresh parsley.

TROFIE AL PESTO

A Ligurian dish featuring trofie pasta served with fresh pesto, a basil-based sauce made with pine nuts, Parmesan, and garlic.

INGREDIENTS

- 1 lb trofie pasta
- 2 cups fresh basil leaves
- 1/4 cup pine nuts
- 1/2 cup Parmesan cheese
- 2 garlic cloves
- Olive oil

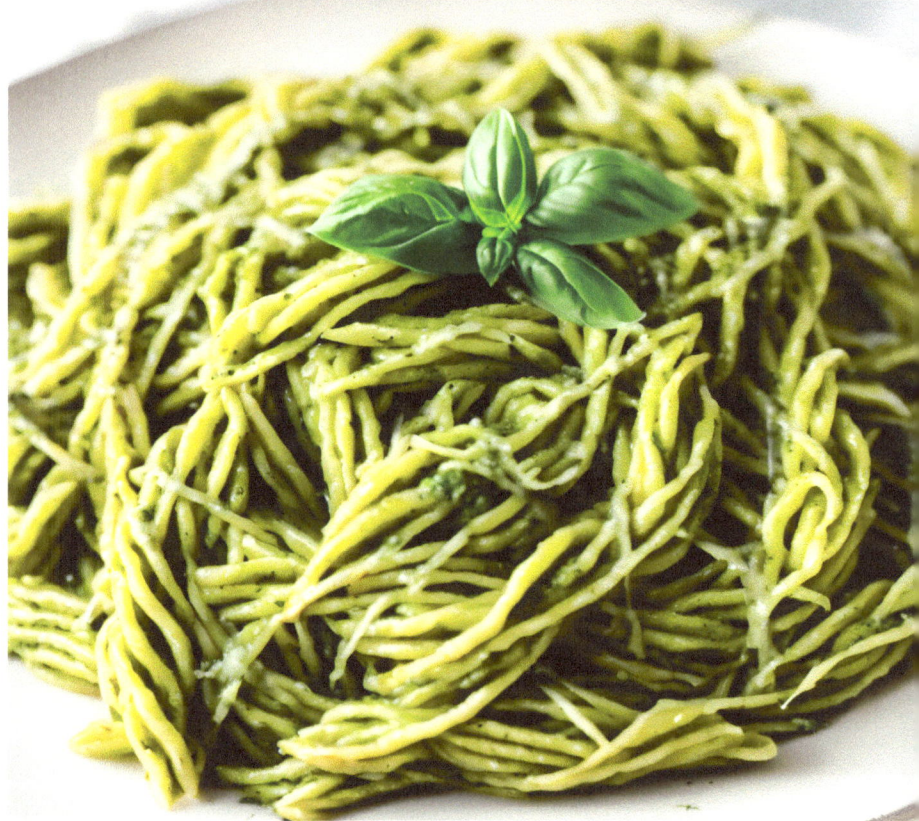

DIRECTIONS

STEP 1

Blend basil, pine nuts, garlic, and Parmesan in a food processor while slowly adding olive oil to form a smooth pesto.

STEP 2

Cook trofie pasta, then toss with the pesto sauce.

STEP 3

Serve with extra Parmesan cheese.

DESSERT

TIRAMISU

Tiramisu is perhaps the most famous Italian dessert worldwide. A delicate, layered dessert made of coffee-soaked ladyfingers, mascarpone cheese, cocoa, and a hint of liquor, traditionally Marsala or rum.

INGREDIENTS

- 6 large egg yolks
- 1 cup sugar
- 1 cup mascarpone cheese
- 1 ½ cups heavy cream
- 2 cups strong brewed coffee, cooled
- 2 tbsp coffee liqueur (optional)
- 2 packs ladyfingers
- Unsweetened cocoa powder for dusting

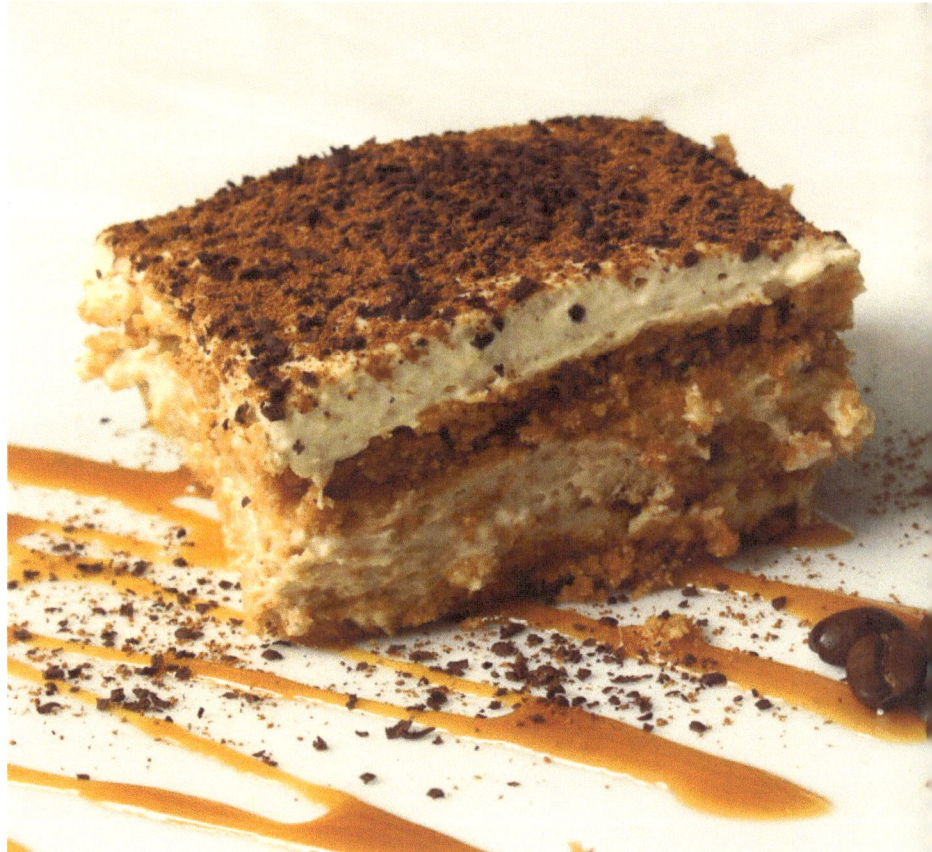

DIRECTIONS

STEP 1

Whisk egg yolks and sugar together until pale and thick.

STEP 2

Fold in mascarpone cheese until smooth.

STEP 3

Whip the heavy cream until stiff peaks form, then gently fold it into the mascarpone mixture.

STEP 4

In a shallow dish, combine coffee and coffee liqueur, and dip the ladyfingers in briefly (don't soak them).

STEP 5

Layer half of the dipped ladyfingers in the bottom of a baking dish, then spread half of the mascarpone mixture on top.

STEP 6

Repeat the layers, finishing with a layer of mascarpone mixture.

STEP 7

Refrigerate for at least 4 hours or overnight. Dust with cocoa powder before serving.

CANNOLI

Cannoli are crispy, tube-shaped pastries filled with a sweet, creamy filling made from ricotta cheese. Often garnished with chocolate chips or candied fruit, they are a staple of Sicilian cuisine.

INGREDIENTS

- 2 cups all-purpose flour
- 2 tbsp sugar
- 2 tbsp cocoa powder
- 1/2 tsp cinnamon
- 2 tbsp butter
- 1 egg, beaten
- 1/2 cup white wine
- 2 cups ricotta cheese
- 1 cup powdered sugar
- 1 tsp vanilla extract
- Chocolate chips for garnish

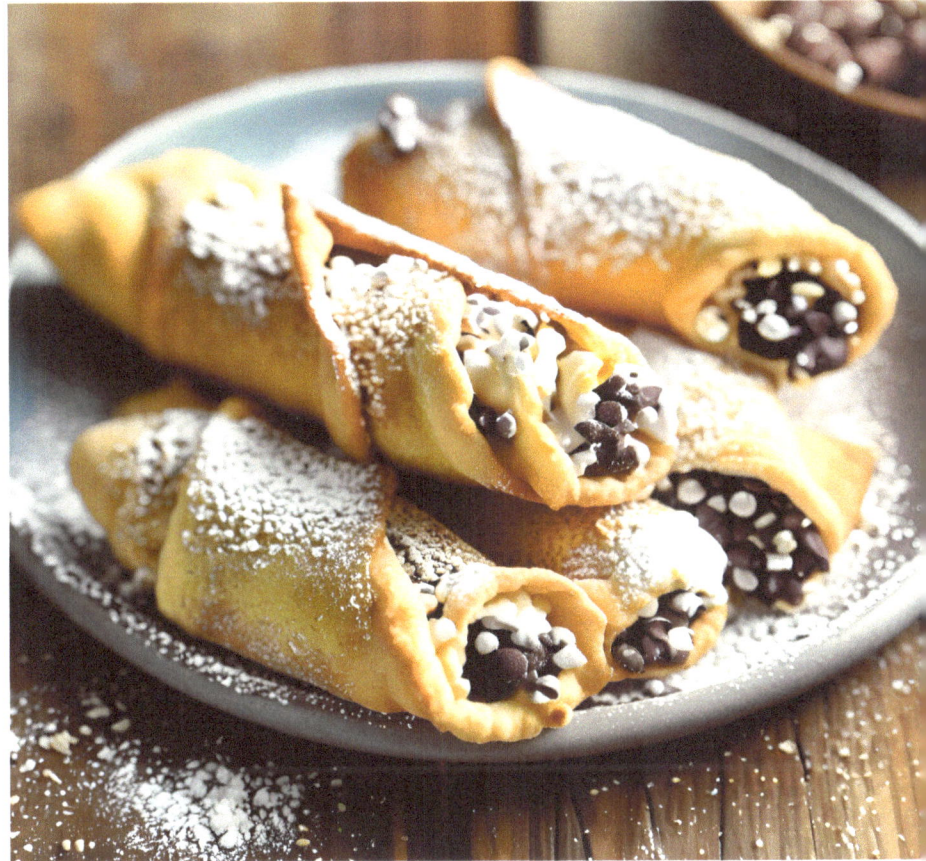

DIRECTIONS

STEP 1
Combine the flour, sugar, cocoa powder, cinnamon, and butter in a food processor. Add egg and wine and pulse until dough forms.

STEP 2
Roll the dough out thinly, cut into circles, and wrap around cannoli tubes. Deep-fry in hot oil until golden.

STEP 3
Drain the shells and allow them to cool.

STEP 4
For the filling, combine ricotta, powdered sugar, and vanilla. Mix until smooth.

STEP 5
Pipe the ricotta filling into the cooled shells and garnish with chocolate chips or candied fruit.

PANNA COTTA

A creamy, chilled dessert originating from the Piedmont region, panna cotta (which means "cooked cream") is made from sweetened cream set with gelatin.

- 2 cups heavy cream
- 1 cup whole milk
- 1/2 cup sugar
- 1 tsp vanilla extract
- 2 tsp gelatin
- 1/4 cup water

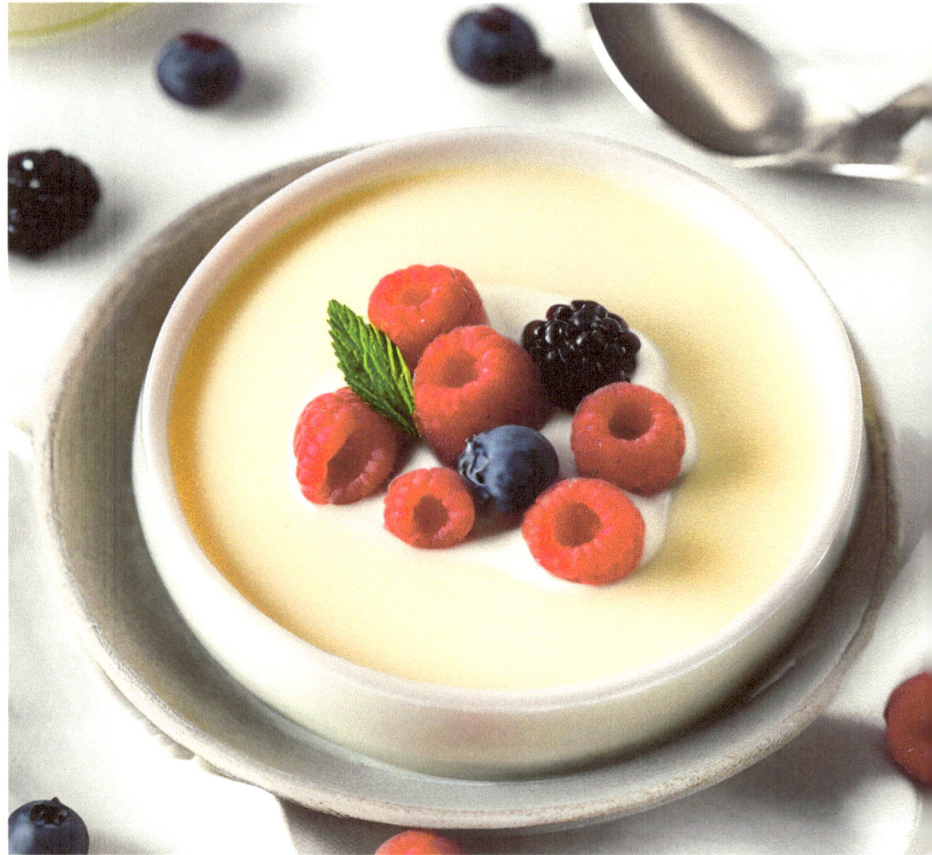

DIRECTIONS

STEP 1

In a saucepan, combine the cream, milk, and sugar over medium heat. Stir until the sugar dissolves and the mixture is hot, but not boiling.

STEP 2

Bloom the gelatin in the water, then stir it into the cream mixture.

STEP 3

Pour the mixture into serving glasses and refrigerate for at least 4 hours until set.

STEP 4

Serve with a berry compote or caramel sauce.

ZABAGLIONE

Zabaglione is a classic Italian custard made with egg yolks, sugar, and Marsala wine, typically served warm over fresh fruit or as a stand-alone dessert.

INGREDIENTS

- 6 large egg yolks
- 1/2 cup sugar
- 1 cup Marsala wine
- Fresh berries for garnish

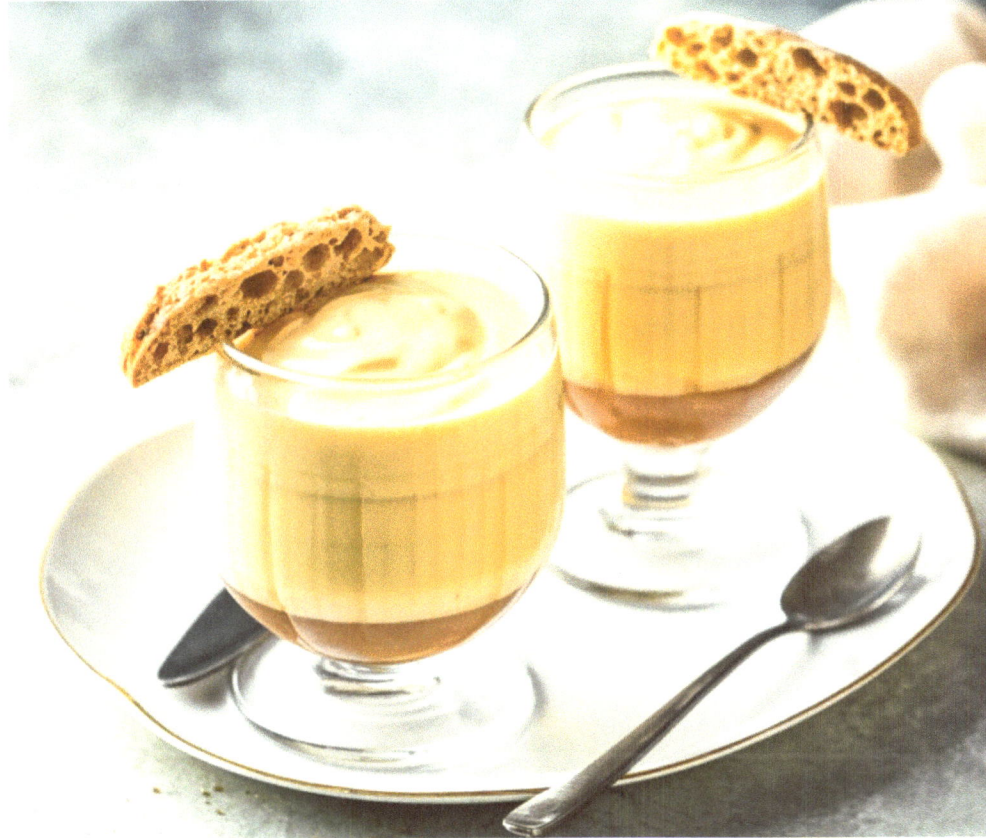

DIRECTIONS

STEP 1

In a heatproof bowl, whisk together the egg yolks and sugar until pale.

STEP 2

Set the bowl over a double boiler, whisking constantly. Gradually add the Marsala wine.

STEP 3

Continue whisking for 8-10 minutes until the mixture thickens and becomes frothy.

STEP 4

Serve immediately over fresh berries or enjoy on its own.

RICOTTA CHEESECAKE

A lighter, fluffier version of traditional cheesecake, this dessert uses ricotta cheese for a softer, creamier texture.

INGREDIENTS

- 2 lbs ricotta cheese
- 1 cup sugar
- 4 eggs
- 1 tsp vanilla extract
- 1 tbsp lemon zest
- 1 ½ cups graham cracker crumbs
- 1/4 cup butter, melted

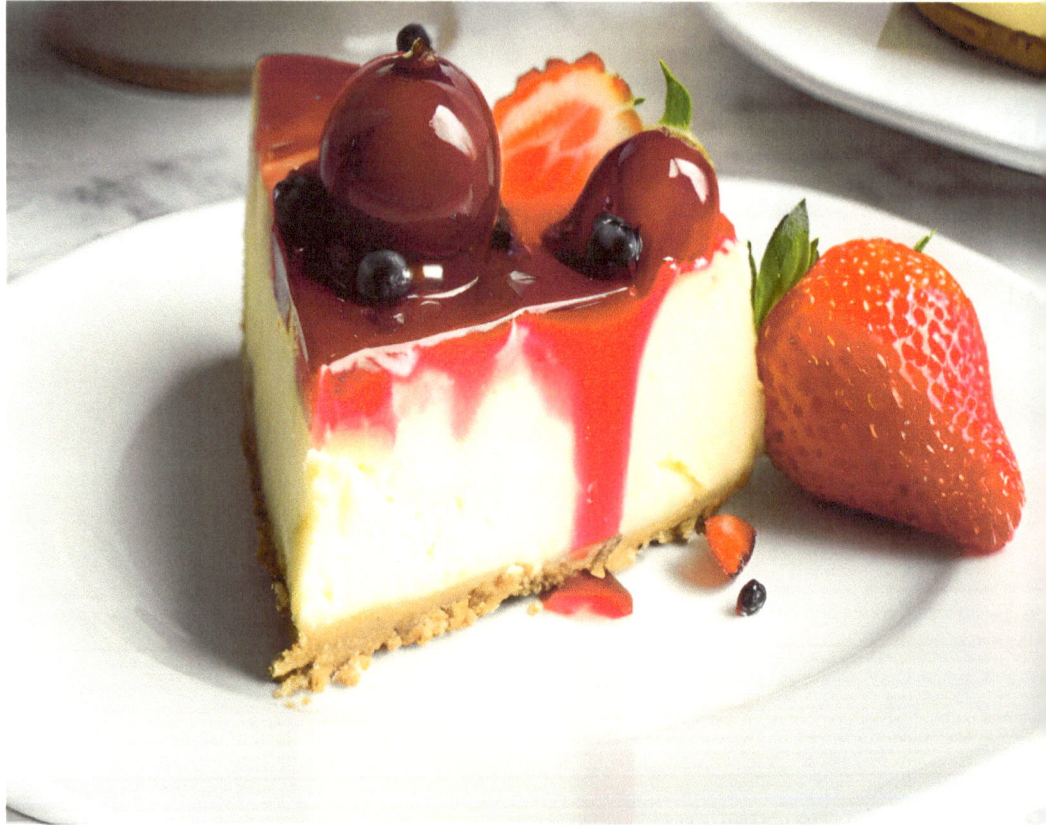

DIRECTIONS

STEP 1

Preheat the oven to 350°F. Combine the graham cracker crumbs and melted butter, pressing them into the bottom of a springform pan.

STEP 2

Beat the ricotta with sugar, eggs, vanilla, and lemon zest until smooth.

STEP 3

Pour the mixture over the crust and bake for 50 minutes, until the center is set.

STEP 4

Let cool completely before serving.

TORTA DELLA NONNA

A Tuscan custard pie topped with pine nuts, Torta della Nonna (Grandmother's Cake) is an iconic Italian dessert that combines a buttery pastry crust with creamy custard filling.

INGREDIENTS

- 2 cups all-purpose flour
- 1/2 cup butter, cubed
- 1/4 cup sugar
- 1 egg yolk
- 1 cup milk
- 1 tbsp flour (for custard)
- 3 egg yolks
- 1/2 cup sugar
- 1 tsp vanilla extract
- Pine nuts for garnish

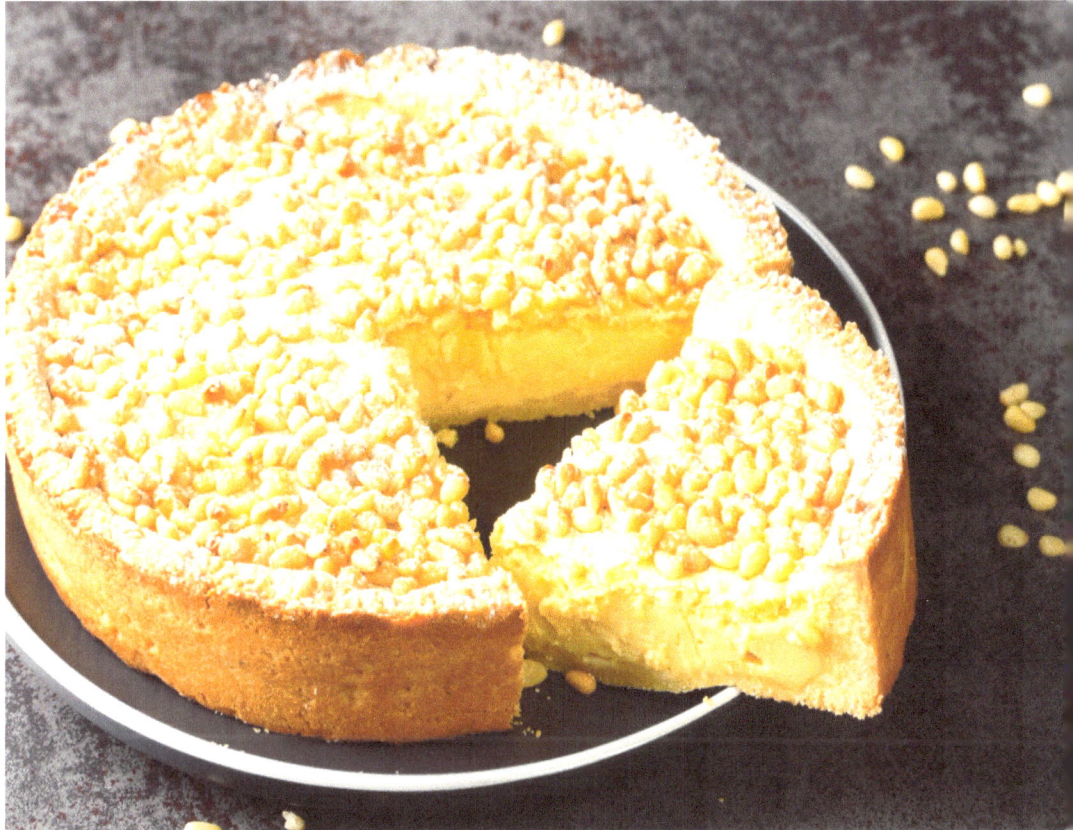

DIRECTIONS

STEP 1

For the crust, combine flour, butter, and sugar, then mix in the egg yolk. Press the dough into a tart pan.

STEP 2

For the custard, heat milk in a saucepan. In a separate bowl, whisk egg yolks, sugar, and flour, then add to the warm milk. Stir until thickened.

STEP 3

Pour the custard into the cooled crust and bake for 25 minutes at 350°F.

STEP 4

Garnish with pine nuts and bake for an additional 5 minutes. Cool before serving.

BISCOTTI DI PRATO

These twice-baked cookies, often referred to as "cantucci," originate from Prato and are traditionally served with Vin Santo wine for dipping.

INGREDIENTS

- 2 cups all-purpose flour
- 1 1/4 cups sugar
- 2 eggs
- 1/2 cup almonds, chopped
- 1/2 tsp baking powder
- 1 tsp vanilla extract

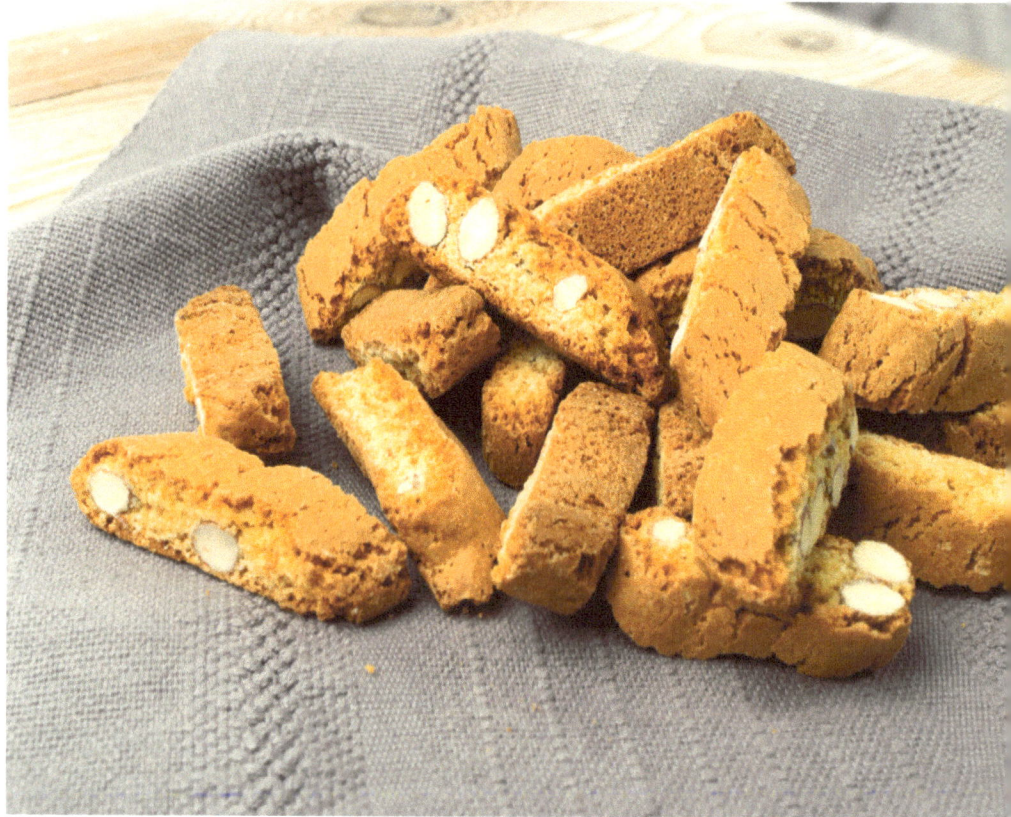

DIRECTIONS

STEP 1

Preheat the oven to 350°F. Mix the dry ingredients and add eggs and vanilla to form a dough.

STEP 2

Shape the dough into a log and bake for 20-25 minutes.

STEP 3

Slice the log into cookies and bake again for 10 minutes until crisp.

CASSATA SICILIANA

This elaborate Sicilian dessert is made with ricotta cheese, candied fruit, and sponge cake, often soaked in liqueur and decorated with icing and chocolate.

INGREDIENTS

- 2 cups ricotta cheese
- 1/2 cup powdered sugar
- 1/2 cup candied orange peel
- 1/4 cup maraschino cherries
- 1 lb sponge cake
- 1/2 cup rum

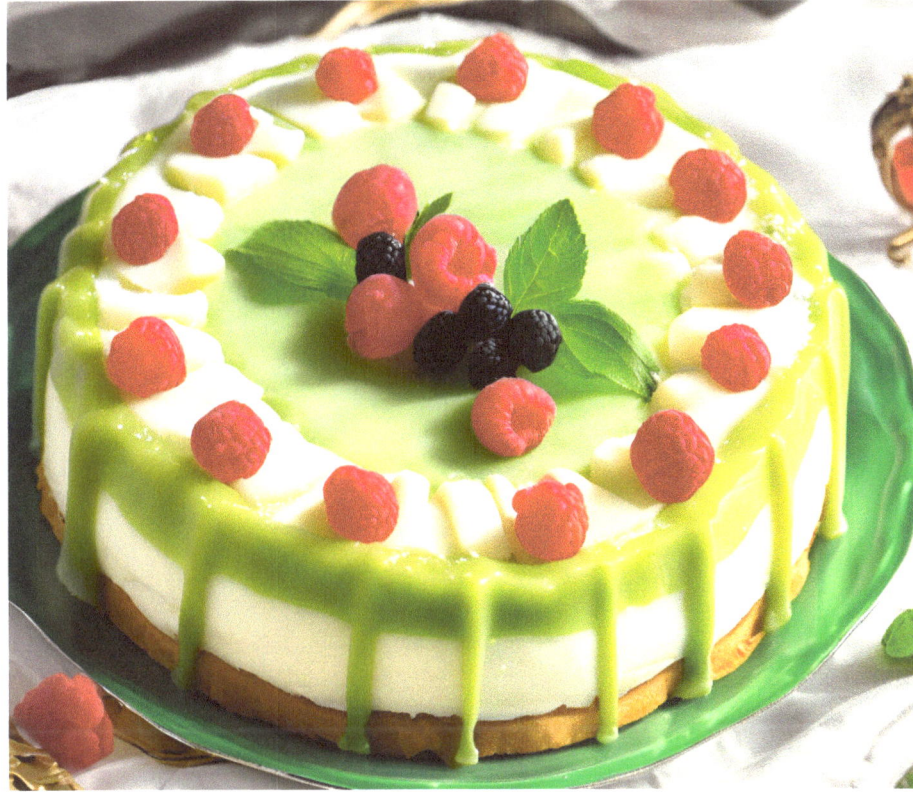

DIRECTIONS

STEP 1

Mix the ricotta with powdered sugar and fold in the candied fruits.

STEP 2

Layer the sponge cake and soak it with rum, then spread the ricotta mixture between the layers.

STEP 3

Chill for a few hours, then cover with icing and garnish with more fruit.

SEMIFREDDO

This frozen Italian dessert is halfway between ice cream and mousse, often flavored with chocolate, fruit, or nuts.

INGREDIENTS

- 3 eggs
- 1/2 cup sugar
- 1 cup whipped cream
- 1/2 cup chocolate chips (or any flavoring)

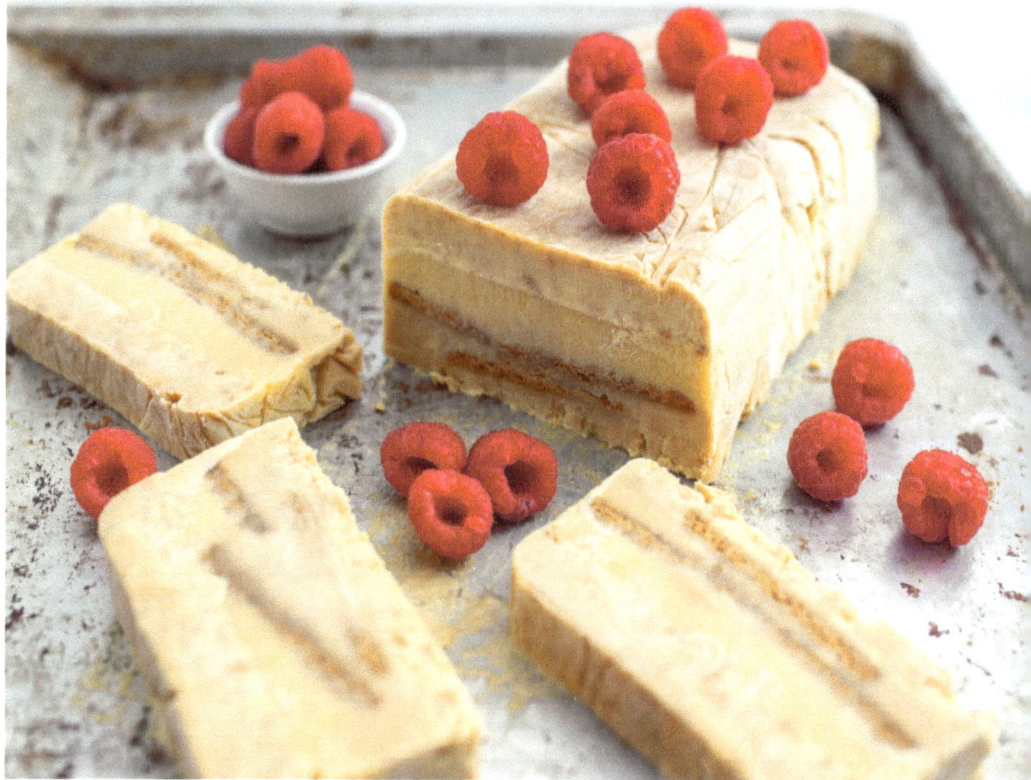

DIRECTIONS

STEP 1

Whisk the eggs and sugar until fluffy, then fold in whipped cream and any flavoring.

STEP 2

Pour into a mold and freeze for at least 4 hours until firm.

PISTACHIO GELATO

A rich, creamy, and nutty version of ice cream, this gelato is made with pistachios for an authentic Italian flavor.

INGREDIENTS

- 1 cup pistachios, shelled
- 2 cups whole milk
- 1 cup heavy cream
- 1/2 cup sugar
- 4 egg yolks

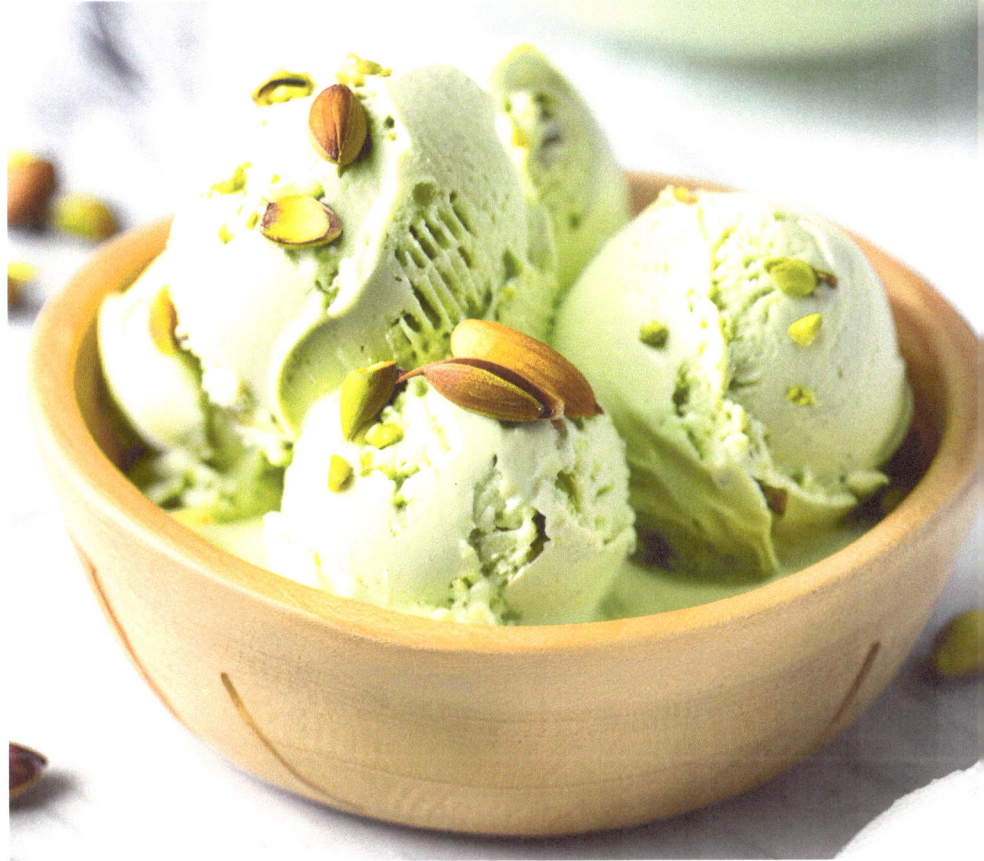

DIRECTIONS

STEP 1

Blend pistachios into a paste, then heat milk, cream, and sugar in a saucepan.

STEP 2

Whisk egg yolks and add them to the warm milk mixture.

STEP 3

Once it thickens, add the pistachio paste and freeze in an ice cream maker.

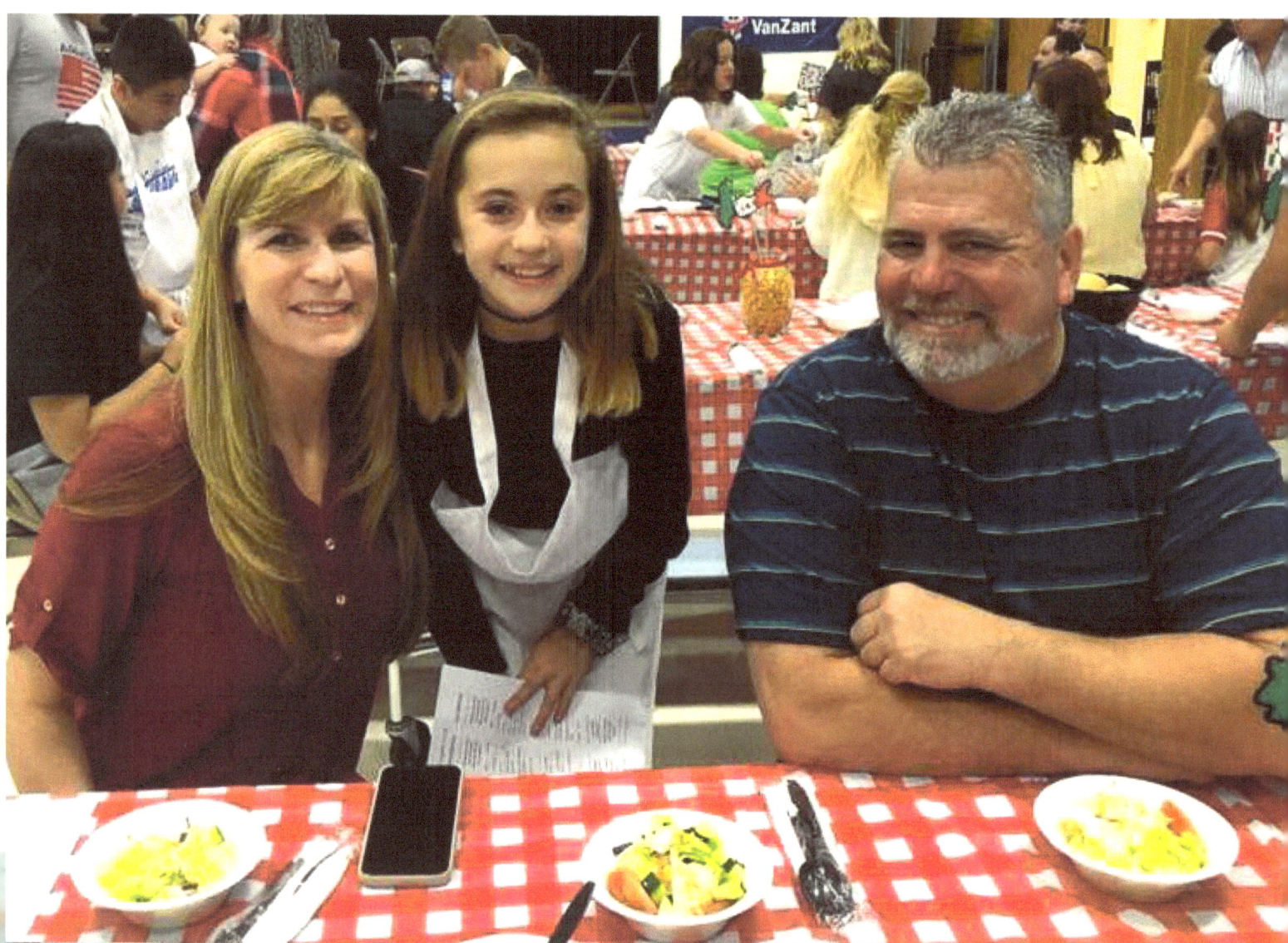
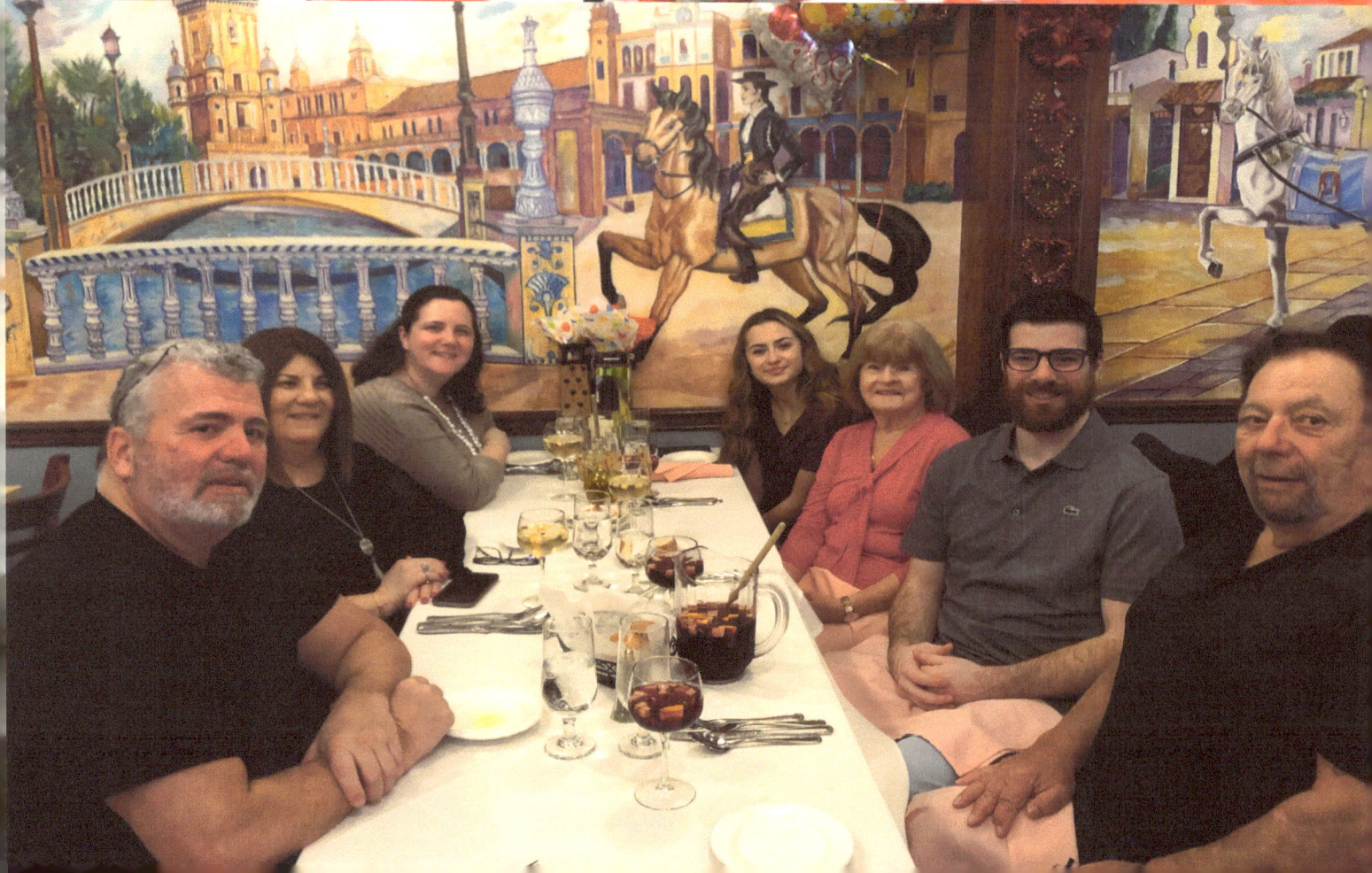

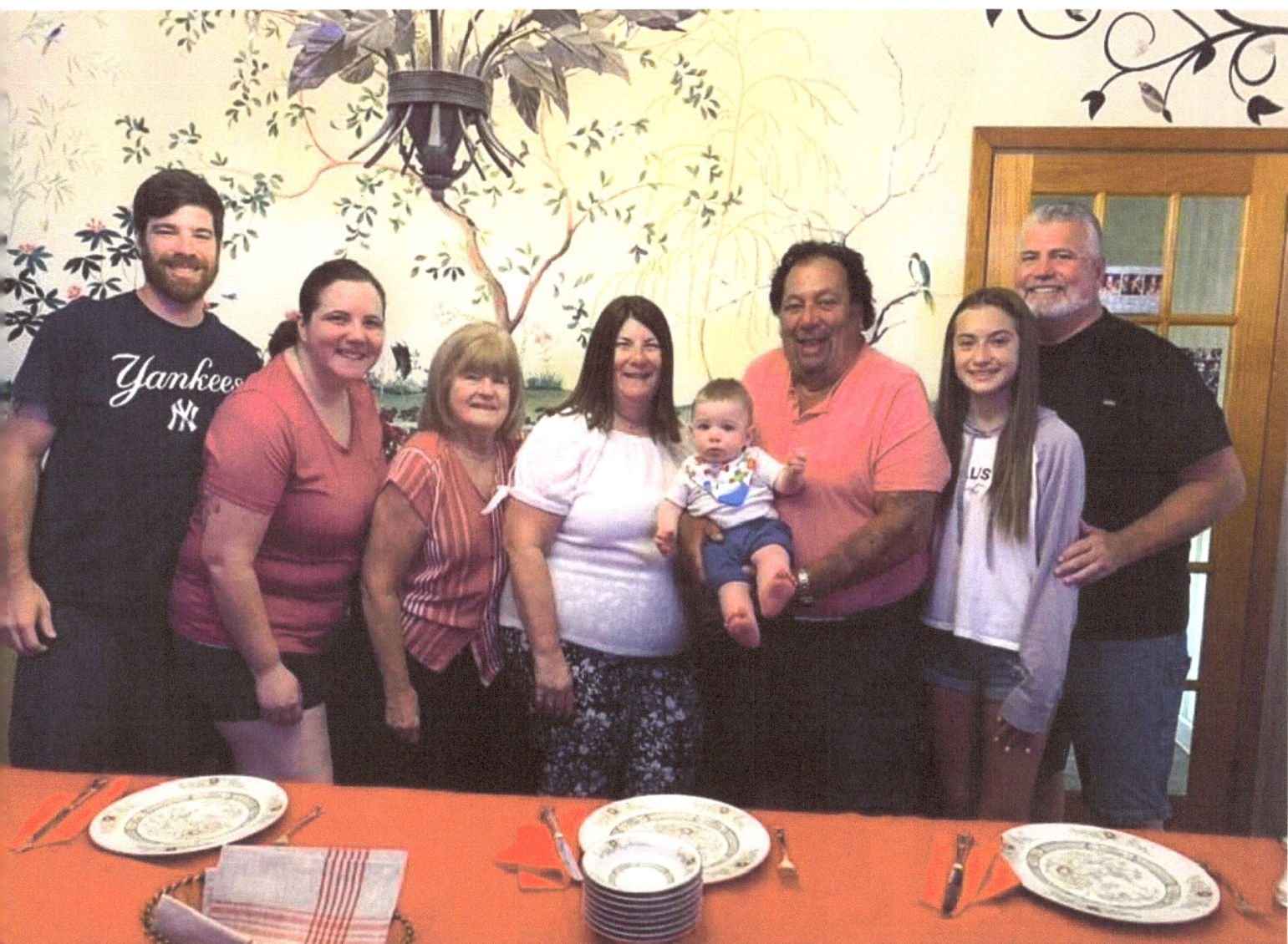
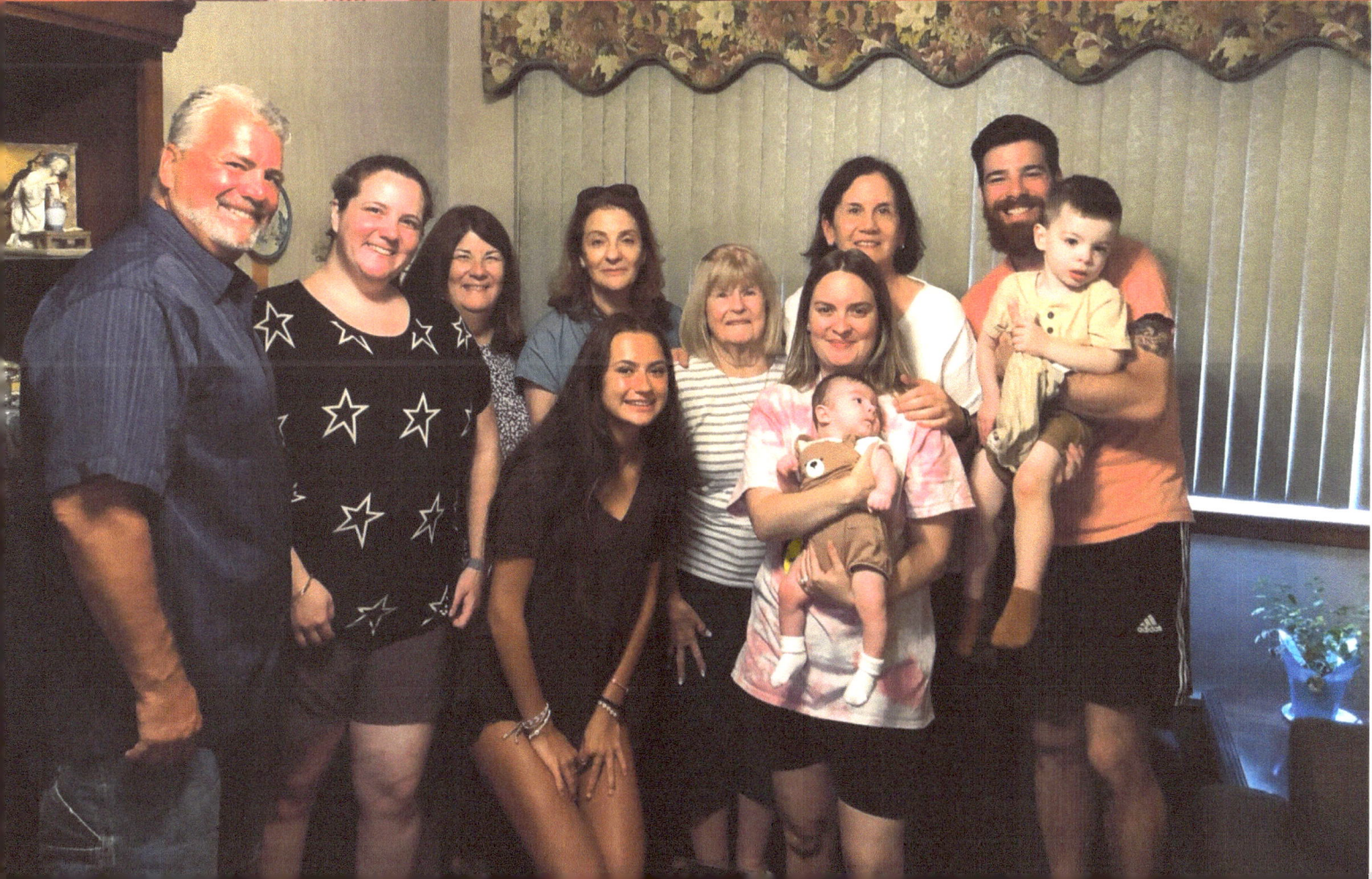

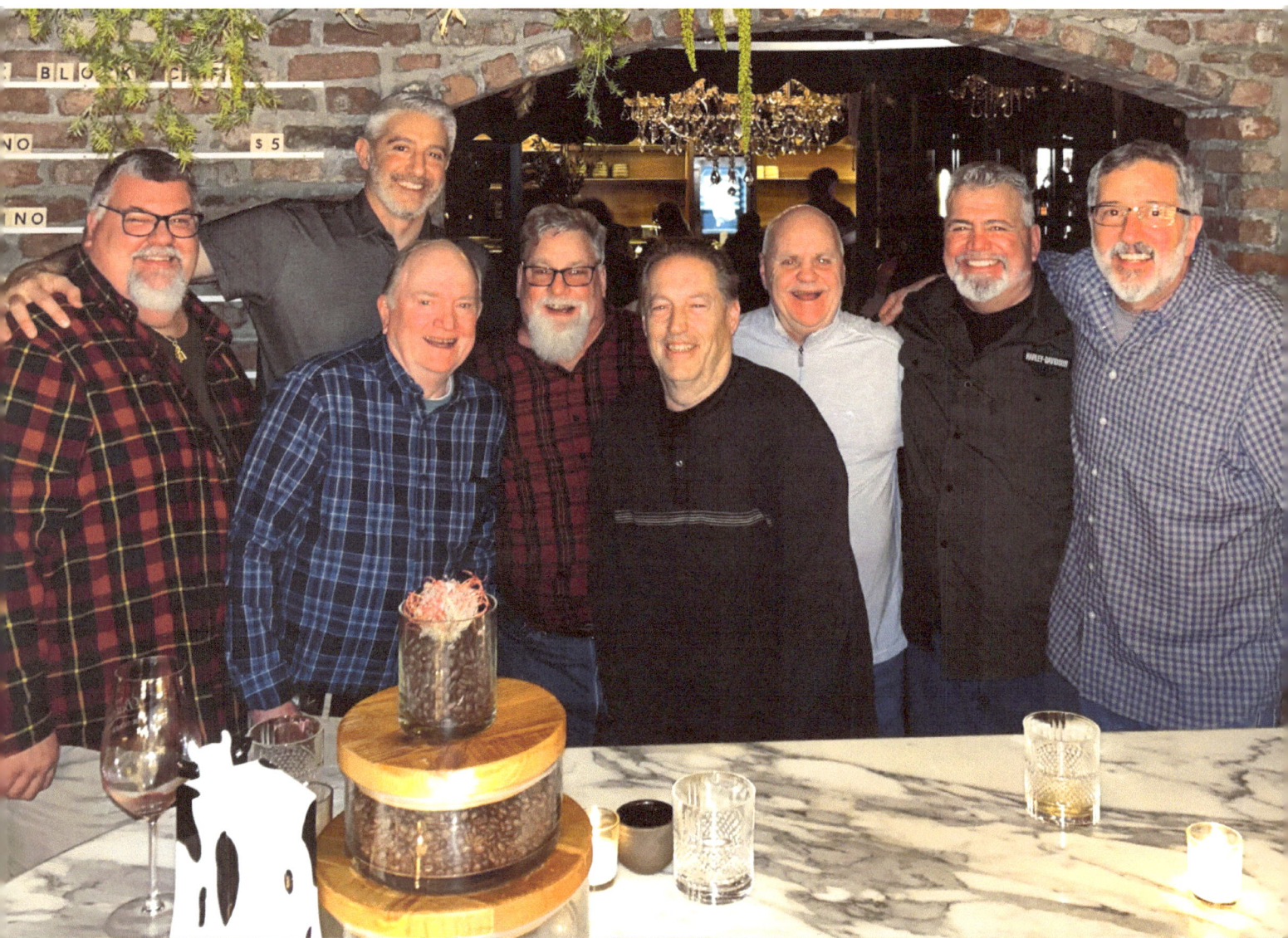
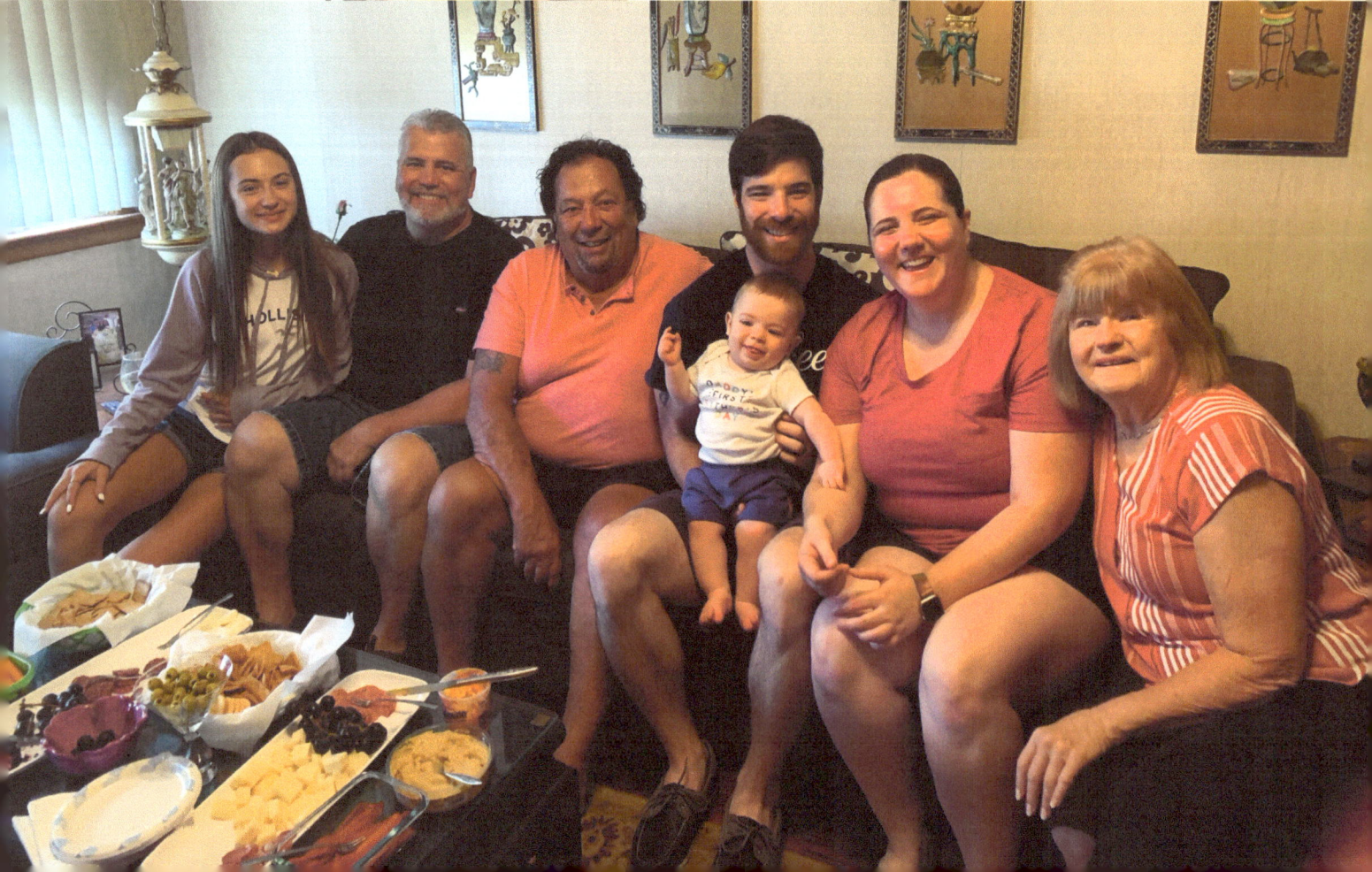

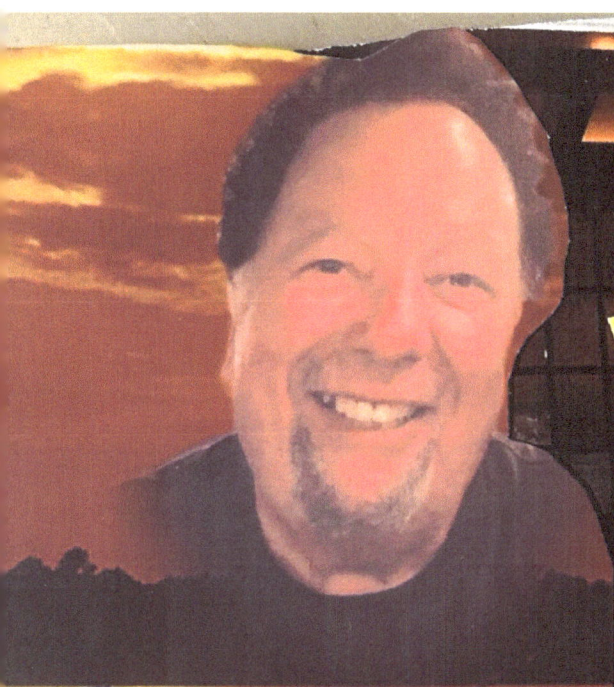

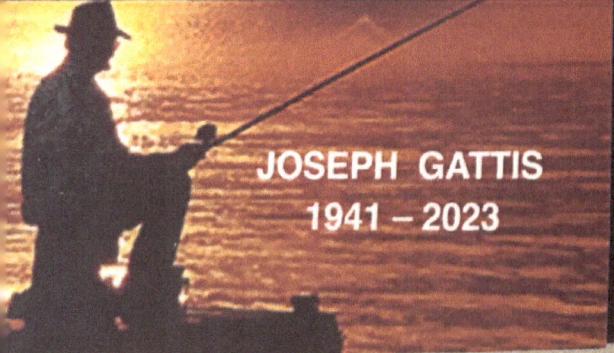

JOSEPH GATTIS
1941 – 2023

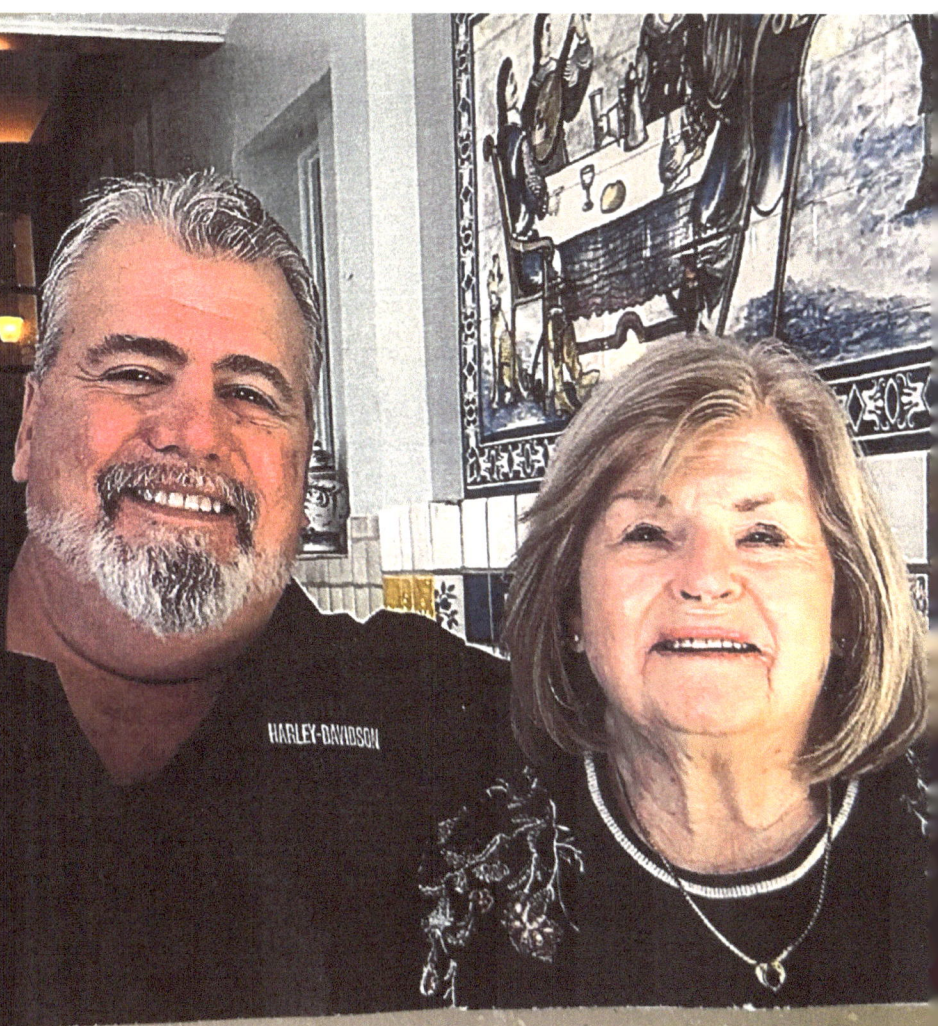

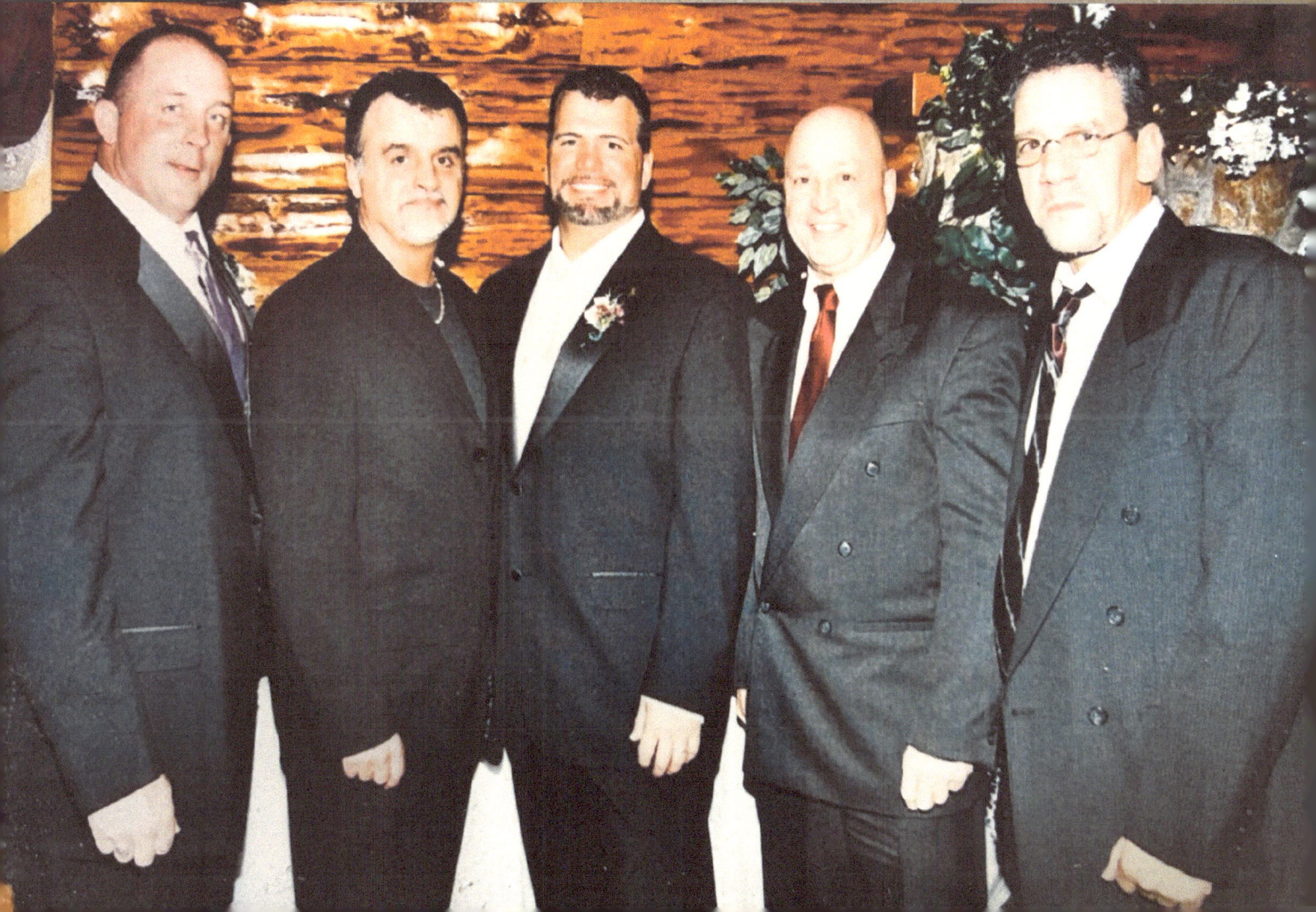

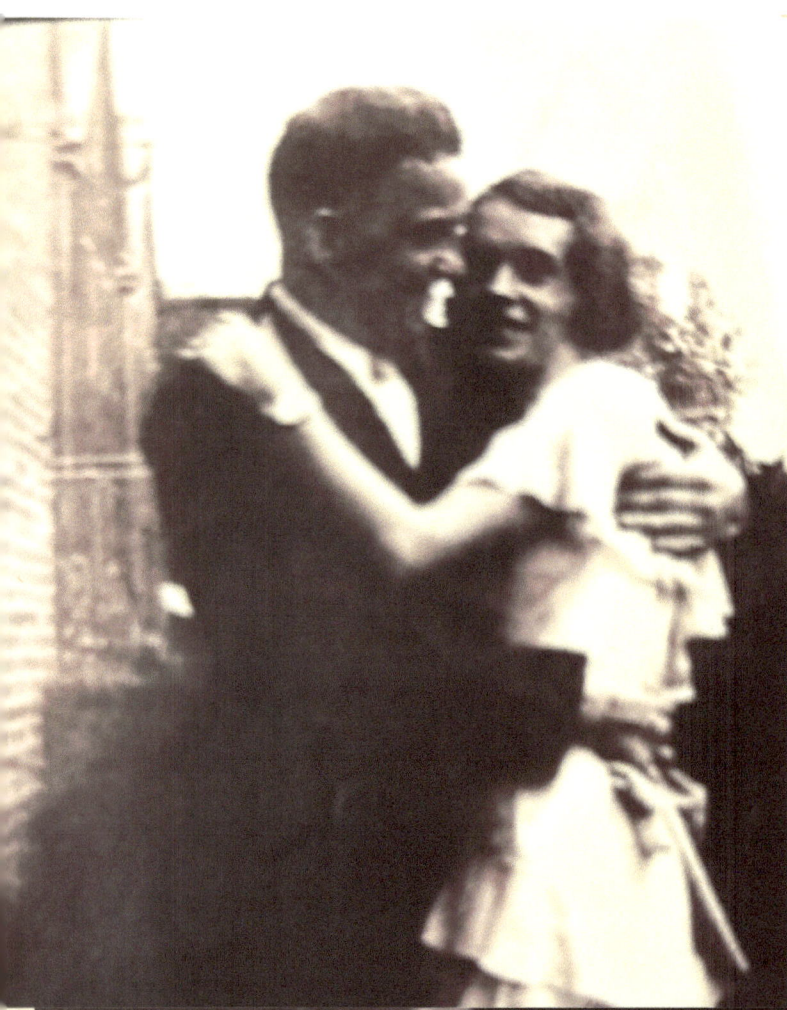

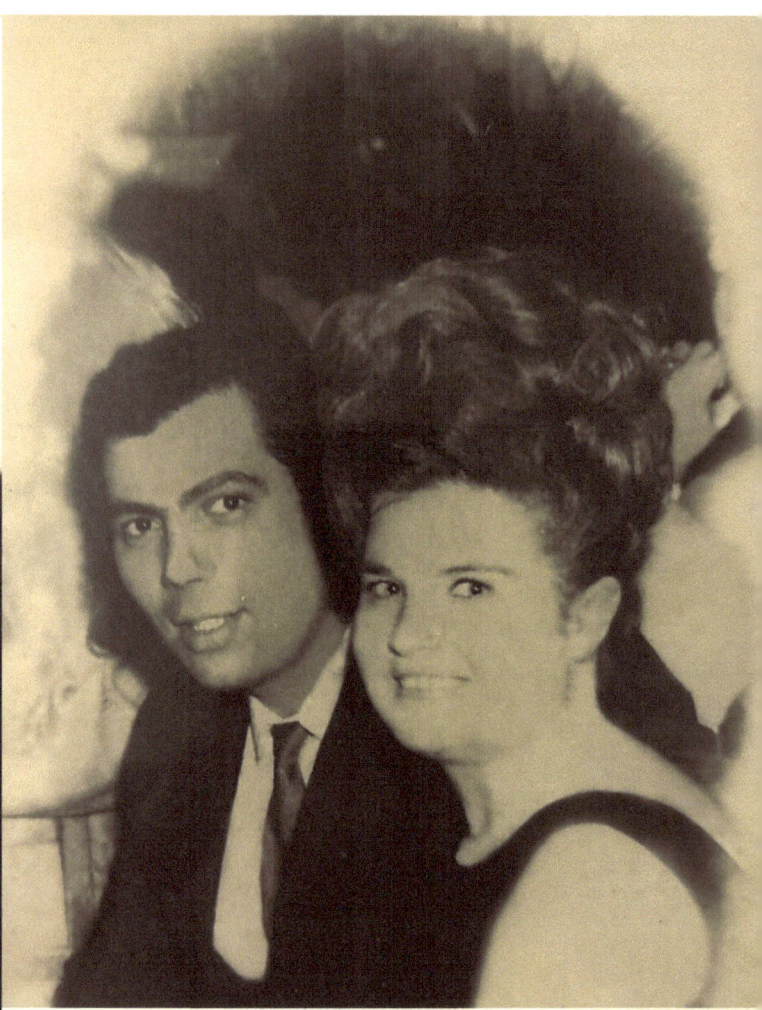

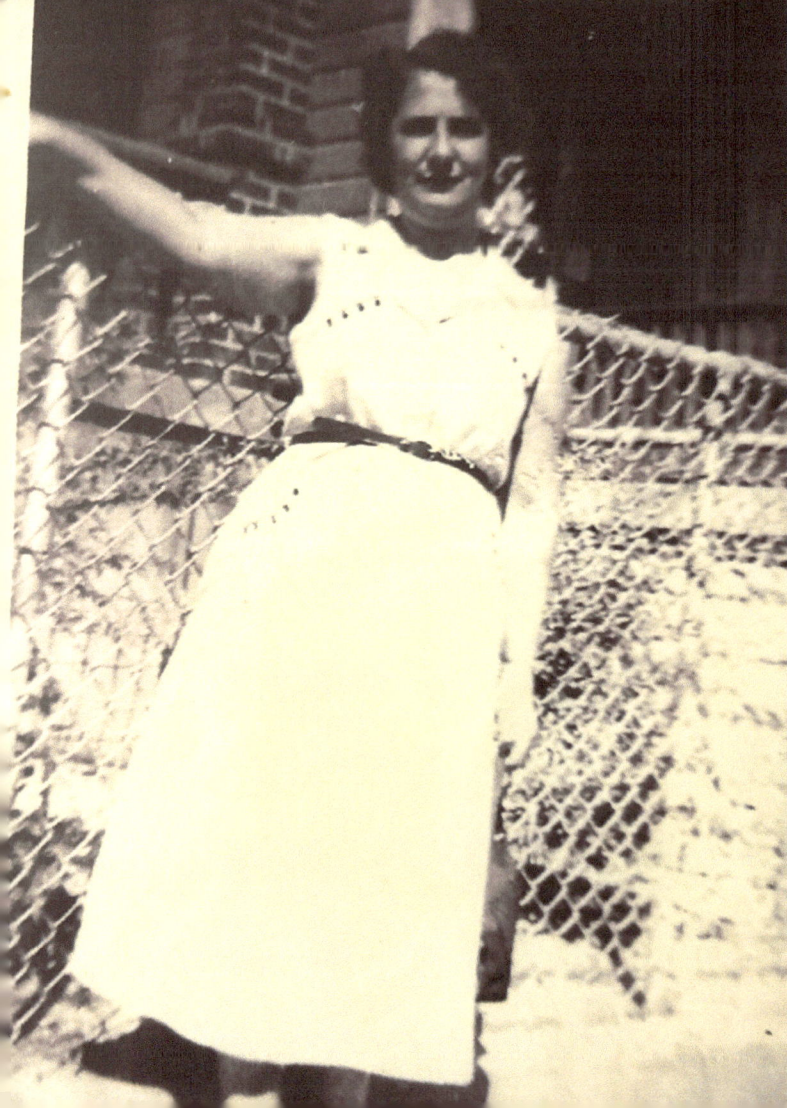

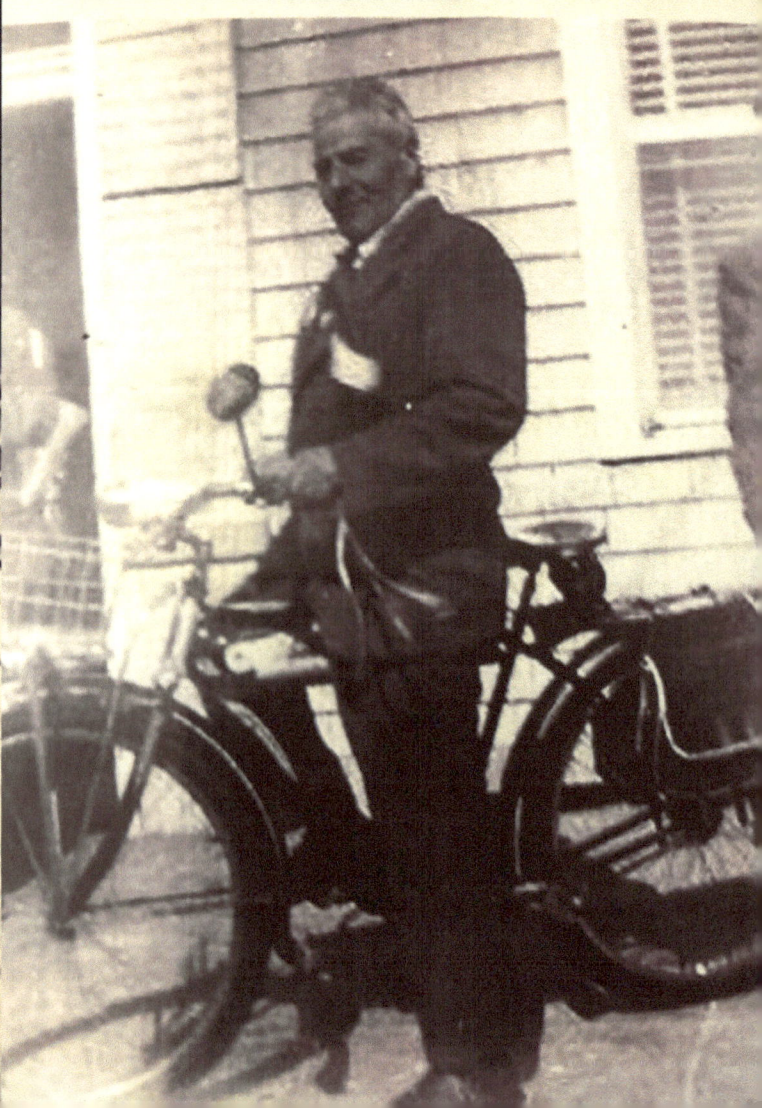

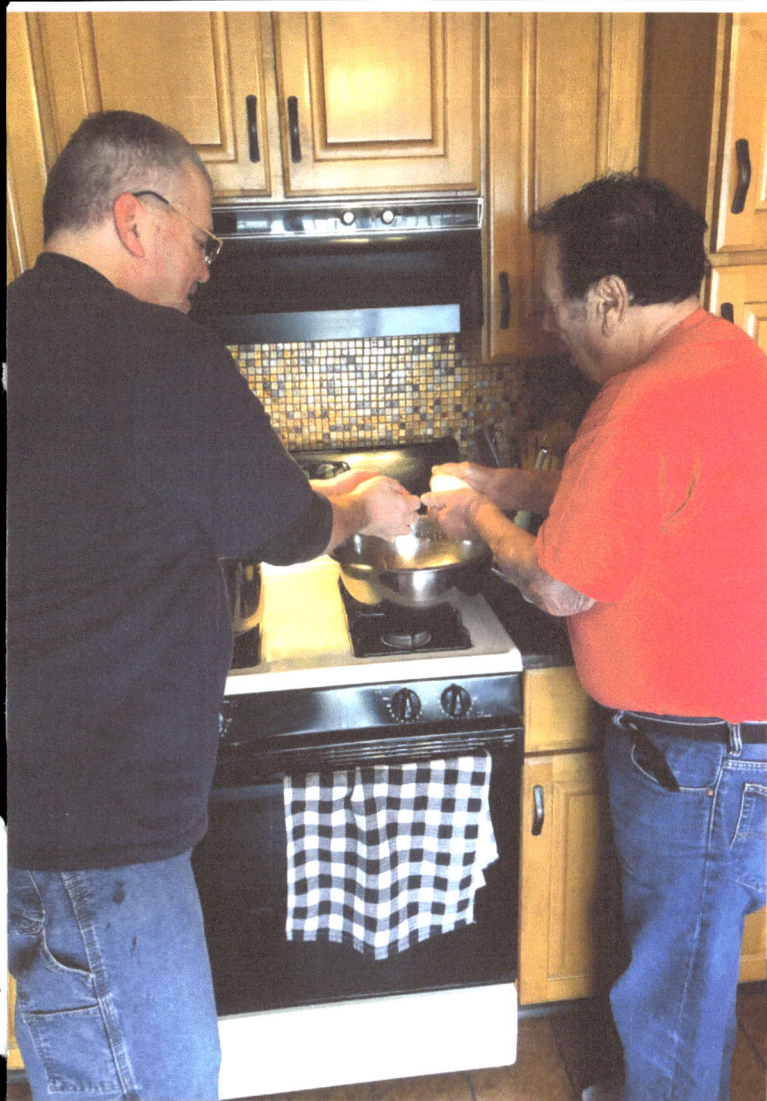
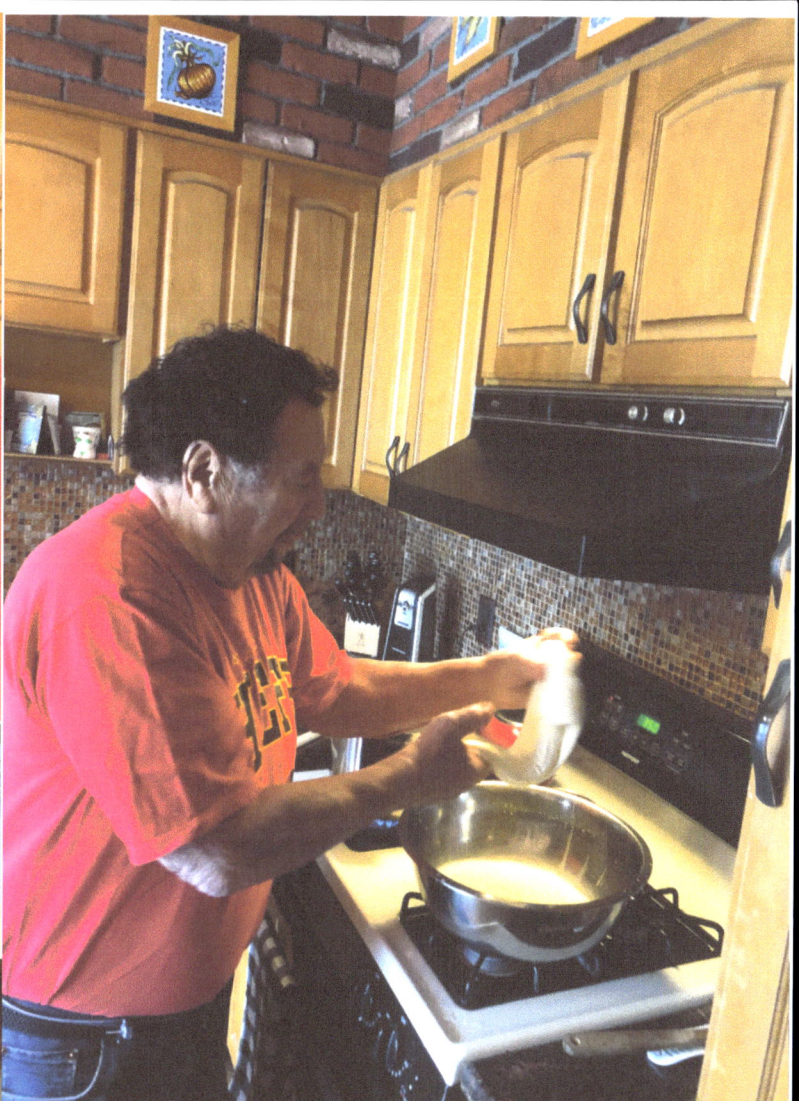
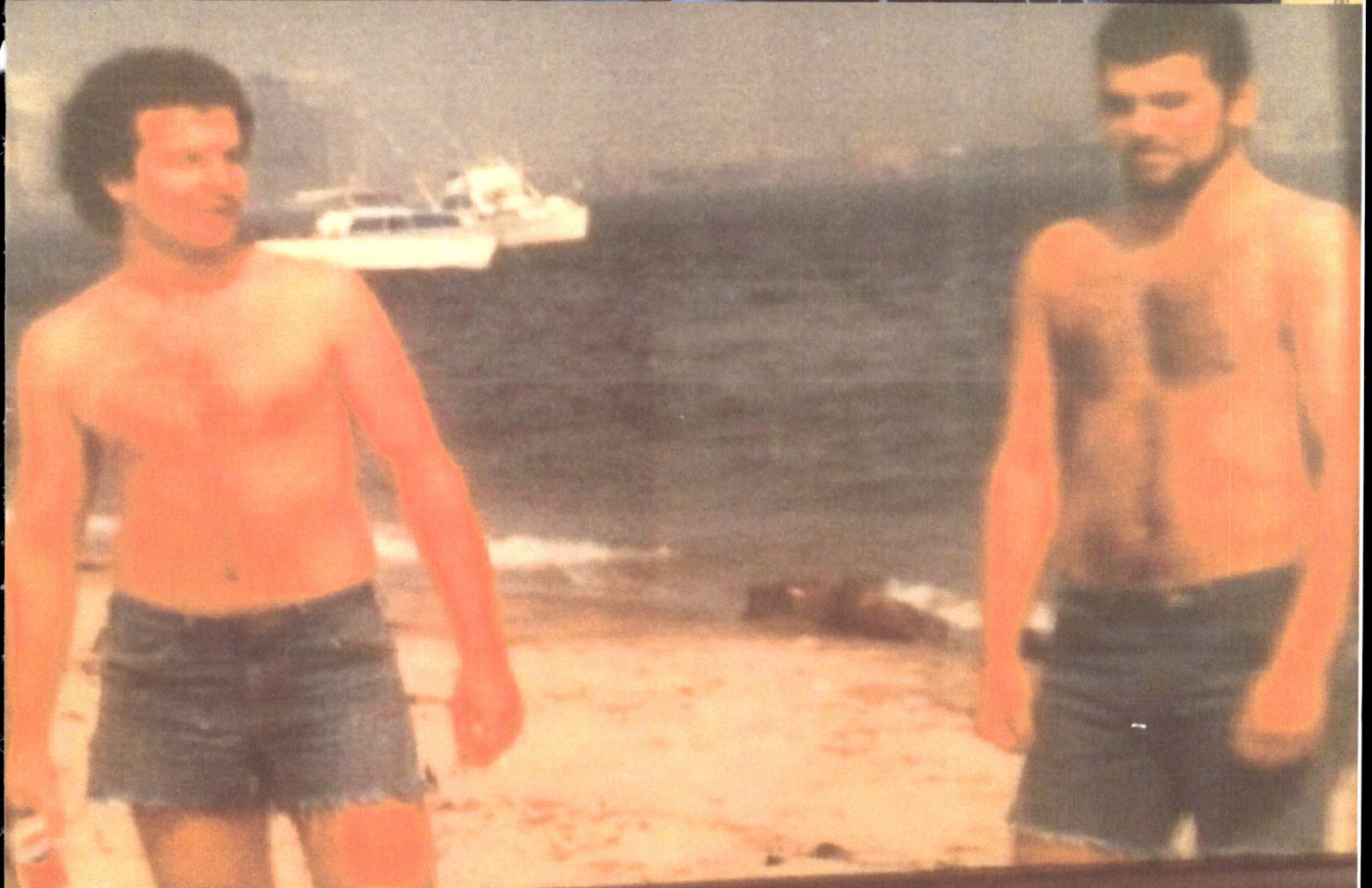